T5-AQR-451

Body Fluids
and Electrolytes

A PROGRAMMED PRESENTATION

Body Fluids and Electrolytes

A PROGRAMMED PRESENTATION

NORMA JEAN WELDY, R.N., B.S., M.S.

Professor of Nursing, Goshen College,
Goshen, Indiana

FIFTH EDITION

with 33 illustrations

The C. V. Mosby Company

ST. LOUIS • WASHINGTON, D.C. • TORONTO   1988

A TRADITION OF PUBLISHING EXCELLENCE

Editor: Don E. Ladig
Assistant editor: Robin Carter
Project manager: Kathleen L. Teal
Manuscript editor: Judith Bange
Design: Gail Morey Hudson
Production: Ginny Douglas

FIFTH EDITION

The C.V. Mosby Company
11830 Westline Industrial Drive, St. Louis, Missouri 63146

Library of Congress Cataloging-in-Publication Data

Weldy, Norma Jean.
  Body fluids and electrolytes.

  Bibliography: p.
  Includes index.
  1. Fluid therapy—Programmed instruction.   2. Water-
electrolyte balance (Physiology)—Programmed instruction.
3. Electrolyte therapy—Programmed instruction.
4. Nursing—Programmed instruction.   I. Title   [DNLM:
1. Body fluids—programmed instruction.   2. Electrolytes
—programmed instruction.   QU 18 W445b]
RM170.W44 1988   612'.01522'077   87-7799
ISBN 0-8016-5401-7

JE/VH/VH   9 8 7 6 5 4 3 2 1   03/C/327

Preface

This text is designed to assist nursing students in overcoming some of the confusion about body fluids and electrolytes. A comprehension of body fluids and electrolytes is essential to understanding many clinical conditions. Nursing students who have a better knowledge of body fluids and electrolytes will give more holistic nursing care to patients. This text is designed for students in nursing who have some basic theoretical knowledge of the biological sciences from their high school curriculum. Students who have had further study of anatomy, physiology, and chemistry will be able to proceed more rapidly through the program. The percentages and laboratory values relate to infants, children, young and middle-aged adults, and elderly persons.

The information is given in sequence, from simple to complex. Each step builds on previous learning. There are written summaries followed by review questions throughout the book. These are presented to help the learner decide when to move on to the next section.

Programmed material does not replace the need for a live teacher, but it does present organized information that students can use to learn at their own rate. The teacher will have to decide how to use this program most effectively. I have found classroom discussion useful after the students have completed the program; I then assign them to care for patients. That is followed by seminar discussion in which they discuss case presentations involving various types of fluid and electrolyte imbalance, the signs and symptoms observed, and the nursing care indicated.

The ultimate objective of the program is to develop in nursing students the ability:

1. To use basic technical terms
2. To recognize the need for an accurate clinical estimate of fluid balance
   a. To measure and record fluid intake and output when indicated
   b. To weigh the patient daily when indicated

3. To identify patients likely to have fluid and electrolyte imbalance and to recognize and report the signs and symptoms
4. To identify patients likely to retain sodium and to recognize and report the signs and symptoms
5. To identify patients likely to lose potassium and to recognize and report the signs and symptoms
6. To recognize and report the signs and symptoms of dehydration
7. To identify patients likely to develop a magnesium imbalance and to recognize and report the signs and symptoms
8. To identify patients likely to develop a calcium imbalance and to recognize and report the signs and symptoms
9. To institute nursing measures to minimize imbalance
    a. To replace fluids and electrolytes
        (1) To encourage and provide oral intake in specific amounts
        (2) To know why fluids are essential
        (3) To measure and record intake and output when indicated
        (4) To provide additional fluid before placing the patient on an order of "nothing by mouth"
        (5) To know how and when to force fluids
        (6) To regulate the flow of parenteral fluids safely
    b. To minimize loss of fluids and electrolytes
        (1) To observe and report loss
        (2) To limit the frequency of irrigations with a nasogastic tube and normal saline solutions
    c. To give medications intelligently

I am especially pleased with the reception of the previous editions and would like to express my appreciation to the many persons who have helped to make the present edition possible. Your questions, comments, and suggestions have been incorporated in this edition. I have discovered that the book is being used as a reference as well as a classroom text. Therefore an index has been included. In this fifth edition I have added information regarding infants, children, and elderly persons throughout the book. Case studies have been included to assist in the application of the material. Several tables along with some illustrations have been added.

Norma Jean Weldy

To the student

This is a program to help you understand the need for balance in body fluids and electrolytes. It will help you learn terms necessary in understanding fluid and electrolyte balance. It will help you understand where fluids and electrolytes are located in the body and how they move. You should gain information on how fluids and electrolytes are lost and how they are replaced both in health and in disease. Through this study, you should learn to recognize the signs and symptoms that indicate imbalance of fluids or electrolytes.

The program will help you learn about some of the laboratory tests that indicate imbalance and some common methods of treating the imbalance. Also, you should learn what is important in giving nursing care to patients who have, or may have, an imbalance in fluids or electrolytes.

Each statement or paragraph is called a frame. At the end of each frame, there is a question with a place for you to respond. The answers are given in the left-hand column. As you work through the program, read carefully and completely formulate your answers to the questions before you look at the answer given. Use the template provided to cover the answer column. If you have questions, consult your instructor.

There are four types of statements to be completed:

1. Sometimes there is a blank to complete the statement. If so, write your answer in the blank and then compare it with the correct response in the answer column.

2. Sometimes you will need to make a choice from two or three answers. Those statements are written as follows:

   This book (will? will not?) help you understand body fluids and electrolytes. Circle the correct choice and compare your response with the answer column.

3. Some statements ask you to respond to questions or situations in your own words. Check your written answer with the suggestions made in the answer

column. Your answer does not have to be identical, but it must contain the same idea.

4. Some statements ask you to select the right answers from a list of several possible answers. Make a check by the correct answers and compare your response with the answer column.

Contents

PART I

Fluid and electrolyte balance

Introduction, 1

Body fluid compartments, 2

Distribution of body fluids, 4

Constituents of body fluids, 6

    Electrolytes, 6

        Summary, 11

        Review, 12

Normal electrolyte composition of the fluid compartments, 12

Movement of fluid in the body, 14

        Summary, 26

        Review, 27

Normal mechanism by which water and electrolytes enter and leave the body, 28

Types of imbalance, 32

    Fluid volume, 32

    Fluid concentration, 32

    Fluid composition, 33

        Summary, 33

        Review, 34

Controls for maintaining fluid and electrolyte balance, 34

Examples of fluid and electrolyte imbalance, 39

    Extracellular fluid volume imbalance, 39

    Extracellular fluid concentration imbalance, 40

    Imbalance in the composition of extracellular fluid, 41

Summary, 42
Review, 42

PART 2

Acid-base balance/   Hydrogen ion concentration, 43
imbalance   Summary, 47
              Review, 47
          Defense mechanisms, 48
              The buffer system, 49
              The respiratory system, 51
              The renal system, 52
              Summary, 55
              Review, 56
          Clinical conditions of imbalance, 56
              Respiratory acidosis, 56
              Respiratory alkalosis, 58
              Metabolic acidosis, 60
              Metabolic alkalosis, 62
              Combination of types of imbalance, 64
              Effects of acidosis and alkalosis on the body, 64
              Summary, 64
              Review, 65
          Nursing care in acid-base imbalance, 66
              Blood gas analysis, 66
              Respiratory acidosis, 68
              Respiratory alkalosis, 70
              Metabolic acidosis, 71
              Metabolic alkalosis, 73
              General nursing responsibilities, 73
              Summary, 75
              Review, 76
          Case studies, 77

PART 3

Fluid volume   Introduction, 81
imbalance   Fluid volume deficit, 82
              Laboratory findings, 83
              Signs and symptoms, 84
              Overhydration, 90
              Summary, 90
              Review, 91

Fluid requirements, 91
Treatment, 94
Fluids by infusion, 94
    Summary, 103
    Review, 103
Fluid volume excess, 104
  Signs and symptoms, 106
Treatment, 108
    Summary, 109
    Review, 110
Fluid volume shifts, 110
    Summary, 112
    Review, 113
Case studies, 113

PART 4

Electrolyte   Introduction, 115
imbalance   Sodium imbalance, 115
    Sodium deficit, 118
      Summary, 122
      Review, 123
    Sodium excess, 124
      Summary, 127
      Review, 127
Case study, 128
Potassium imbalance, 128
    Potassium deficit, 132
      Summary, 138
      Review, 139
    Potassium excess, 139
      Summary, 143
      Review, 144
Case study, 144
Magnesium imbalance, 145
  Magnesium deficit (hypomagnesemia), 148
      Summary, 157
      Review, 157
    Magnesium excess, 158
      Summary, 160
      Review, 161
Calcium imbalance, 161

Calcium deficit, 166
  Summary, 171
  Review, 172
Calcium excess (hypercalcemia), 172
  Summary, 178
  Review, 179

Bibliography, 180

Body Fluids
and Electrolytes

A PROGRAMMED PRESENTATION

PART 1 Fluid and electrolyte balance

INTRODUCTION

People cannot live without body fluid. Water is the largest single constituent of the body. In the average young to middle-aged adult the total body fluid amounts to about 60% of the body weight, and in a newborn infant 70% to 75% of the total body weight is fluid. By the age of 2 years, the percent of body weight that is fluid is approximately the same as that of a young to middle-aged adult, 60%. In the elderly, because of changes in body tissues, the total body fluid drops to 45% to 50% of body weight. Because of the high percentage of body weight that is fluid, in infants, fluid balance is extremely important. Since the elderly have a much lower percentage of body weight that is fluid, they are also highly likely to develop fluid imbalance. When a person vomits, he loses some of the normal fluid content of the body. If the vomiting continues and he does not drink fluids, the loss may become serious. The person becomes lethargic, the mucous membranes become dry, and the body temperature increases. A person becomes very uncomfortable when the body's fluid content is less than normal.

A loss of 20% of the fluid content is *fatal*. For example, a person with third-degree burns over a major area of the body will lose fluid through seepage from the burned areas. If the fluid is not replaced, he will die. By replacing the body fluid, the nurse can make the person more comfortable and may save his life.

1 From a study of anatomy and physiology we know that body fluids have two main functions. One of the functions of body fluids is to provide transportation of nutrients to the cells and carry waste products from the cells.

transportation of nutrients
and waste products

One function of body fluids is _____

_____.

2 A second major function of body fluids is to provide a medium in which chemical reactions can occur.

Body fluids provide for transport of nutrients and waste products, and they are also necessary so that

chemical reactions

_____ can occur.

BODY FLUID COMPARTMENTS

3 Body fluids are contained within three compartments. These compartments are not bladders tucked away somewhere, but the term "compartment" is a convenient abstraction used to describe where fluid is found in the body. Most of the body fluids are inside the cells, and we call this the intracellular compartment. *Intra-* is a prefix meaning within, or on the inside. When we give intramuscular injections, we give the medication within, or inside, the muscle.

intracellular

The largest amount of body fluids is within the cell and is called _____.

4 The fluid in each cell has its own unique composition, but the concentration of intracellular constituents is similar from one cell to another cell. If you have three kinds of cookies, each cookie may contain different ingredients; but even though they are not alike in composition, we call each of them a cookie, or three cookies. Although the intracellular fluid of individual cells differs in chemical composition, it is similar in concentration. Therefore the intracellular fluid of all the different cells may be considered one large fluid compartment, even though it is contained in individual cells.

a The concentration of constituents in each cell is (the same? similar? different?).

similar

composition

b Each cell has its own chemical _____.

2

5 We may use the term *extracellular* to refer to all the fluid outside the cells. The prefix *extra-* means outside of. In school we participate in extracurricular activities. Extracurricular activities are those pursuits that are not a part of the student's course of study but are important for learning. Extracellular means outside the cell.

intracellular

extracellular

a Fluid that is *within* the cell is called _____.
b Fluid that is *outside* the cell is called _____.

6 The *extracellular* fluid is outside the cell, but part of that fluid is within the blood vessels.

Since *intra-* means within and *-vascular* means vessel, the fluid that is within blood vessels is called

intravascular

_____.

7 Although some of the extracellular fluid is within the blood vessels (intravascular), the rest of the extracellular fluid is between the cells. Since this fluid is *between* the cells and blood vessels, it is called *interstitial* fluid.

Therefore the extracellular fluid is divided into two parts:

intravascular

interstitial

a (within blood vessels) _____
b (between cells) _____

8 If we divide all body fluid into only two groups, we use the cell as our point of reference; so fluids are either inside the cell or outside the cell.

The two main compartments for body fluids are

intracellular

extracellular

a (inside the cell) _____
b (outside the cell) _____

9 We can then divide the extracellular fluids into two groups, those within the blood vessels and those between the cells.

intravascular

interstitial

The former group is called _____, and the latter _____.

10 The fluid compartments are separated by semipermeable membranes. Since the fluids outside the cells (intravascular and interstitial) are constantly mixing through the capillary walls, the extracellular fluid is contained within a communicating chamber.

mixing

The extracellular fluids are (mixing? separate?).

3

11 Label the body fluid compartments in the blanks at the left of the diagram.

Extracellular
Intracellular
Interstitial
Intravascular

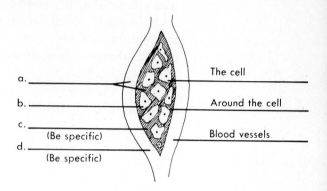

a. _____

b. _____

c. _____
(Be specific)

d. _____
(Be specific)

The cell

Around the cell

Blood vessels

DISTRIBUTION OF BODY FLUIDS

12 Study the figure below and answer the following questions:

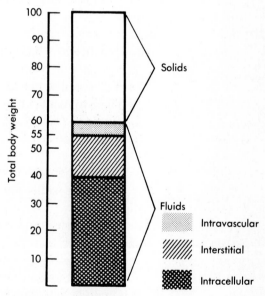

% Body weight in children and young
to middle-aged adults

60%
40

a The percent of total body weight that is fluid is ____.
b The fluid inside the cells is ____% of body weight.

c The fluid within the blood vessels is _____% of body weight.

13 Newborn infants have a higher proportion of body weight that is fluid than do children and adults. Up to age 2 years, the proportion of body weight that is fluid is from 70% to 75%.

In infants the percent of total body weight that is fluid

70% to 75%   is _____.

14 In infants the percent of fluid inside the cell is 40% of body weight, the same as in young to middle-aged adults. In infants the extracellular fluid is approximately 35% of body weight.

The percent of total body weight that is extracellular

35%   fluid in infants is approximately _____.

15 With age, the total body water diminishes. In the elderly the intracellular fluid is reduced because of tissue loss. The percent of total body weight that is fluid may be reduced to 45% to 50% in persons over age 65.

A person aged 65 is likely to have (45%? 60%? 75%?)

45%   of body weight that is fluid.

16 The body must have fluid to continue its normal processes. The kidneys excrete the largest quantity of fluid, but fluid also leaves the body through the gastrointestinal tract, lungs and skin.

Fluid normally leaves the body through the gastroin-

kidneys   testinal tract, lungs, skin, and _____.

17 The fluid in the body is replenished in two ways. The most obvious is by the ingestion of liquids; but, in addition, meats and vegetables contain 60% to 97% water. Also, the breakdown of food yields water of oxidation. (Water is one of the products of metabolism.) About 10 ml of water is released by the metabolism of each 100 calories of fat, carbohydrate, or protein.

Two sources of fluid for the body are ingestion of liquids and the water in foods. The third source of fluids is

metabolism (water of   by _____.
oxidation)

Electrolytes

18 The body fluids consist of water and dissolved substances. Some substances such as glucose, urea, and creatinine do not dissociate in solution. That is, they do not separate from their complex form into simpler substances when they are in a solution.

does not

Glucose (does? does not?) dissociate when in solution.

19 Although some substances do not dissociate when in solution, other substances do dissociate. For example, when sodium chloride (NaCl) is in a solution, it dissociates, or separates, into two parts or elements.

Some

(Some? All?) substances dissociate when in solution.

20 Before further discussion of body fluid constituents, we shall consider some of the terms being used. Remember: an *atom* is the smallest particle of an element that still has the properties of the element. When two or more atoms combine to form a substance, this is called a *molecule*. Atoms are composed of particles. The particles of an atom are the *proton*, *neutron*, and *electron*. The proton carries a positive charge, the electron carries a negative charge of the same magnitude, and the neutron is neutral.[11] You can remember that the neutron is neutral because "neutron" and "neutral" begin with the same five letters. You can remember that the proton carries a positive charge because both "proton" and "positive" begin with the letter "p." That leaves only the electron to remember as being different.

negative

a The electron of an atom carries a (positive? negative? neutral?) charge.

positive

b The proton of an atom carries a (positive? negative? neutral?) charge.

21 The proton and neutron are in the nucleus, or center, of the atom.

Therefore the nucleus is positively charged because it contains both the neutron, which is neutral, and the

proton

(proton? electron?), which is positive.

22 Electrons carry negative charges and revolve around

the nucleus. As long as the number of electrons in an atom is the same as the number of protons, there is no net charge on the atom (i.e., it is neither positive nor negative). However, atoms may gain, lose, or share electrons and then no longer be neutral.

If an atom either gains or loses electrons, it is no

neutral   longer _____.

23 When an atom carries an electrical charge because it has either gained or lost electrons, we call it an *ion*. An ion is an electrically charged atom or group of atoms.

An atom that has an electrical charge is called a/an

ion   _____.

24 An ion may carry either a positive or a negative charge. When an ion carries a positive charge, it is called a *cation*.

A cation is an ion with a (positive? negative?) elec-

positive   trical charge.

25 Another way to explain an ion with a positive charge, or a cation, is that this ion is an electron donor. It has given away, or lost, electrons. The result is fewer electrons than protons. Since the protons carry the positive charge and the electrons the negative charge, and this ion has given away electrons, the result is a positive charge.

A cation carries a positive electrical charge because

electrons   it has given away _____.

26 It may help you to remember that cations are positive ions if you see that "cation" has a "t" (or +) in it. A cation is an ion that carries a positive electrical charge. However, not all ions are cations. Some ions carry a negative electrical charge. When an ion has gained, or taken on, electrons, it assumes a negative charge. Since the electrons are negatively charged, and we have now added electrons, the result is a negatively charged ion.

gained   Negatively charged ions have (gained? lost?) electrons.

27 An ion that has gained electrons and therefore carries a negative charge is called an anion.

7

a An ion carries a _____ electrical charge.
b A cation carries a _____ electrical charge.

28 Another term we shall use is *electrolyte*. When a substance is dissolved in solution and some of its molecules split or dissociate into electrically charged atoms, or ions, we call that substance an electrolyte. If we take an electrolyte such as sodium chloride (NaCl) and dissolve it in solution, it will dissociate into sodium (Na^+) and chloride (Cl^-).

Sodium is the cation because it carries a positive charge. Chloride carries a negative charge and is called the _____.

anion

29 Electrolytes are the substances we have been discussing that dissociate in solution into electrically charged atoms called _____.

ions

30 An electrolyte dissociates into electrically charged ions when in solution. Therefore, when an electrolyte is dissolved in water, it conducts an electrical current. We can demonstrate this by placing two electrodes in an electrolyte solution and connecting them to a bulb and battery. The dissociation of the electrolyte into charged atoms or ions will conduct an electrical current between the electrodes. The anion, the negatively charged ion, will migrate to the anode, which is the electrode with a positive charge. Remember: positive charges attract negative charges, whereas like charges repel. Therefore the negative ion (anion) will be attracted to the anode.

The anion ($-$) will be attracted to the (positive? negative?) electrode.

positive

31 The positive electrode is called the *anode*, and anions ($-$) will migrate to it. The negative electrode is called the *cathode*, and cations ($+$) will be attracted to it.

The cation is the (positive? negative?) ion.

positive

32 The cation is the positive ion and will be attracted to the cathode.

Therefore the cathode is the (positive? negative?) electrode.

negative

33 Those ions that carry a positive charge are called *cations* (+) and are attracted to the cathode (−) when electricity passes through a solution. The ions carrying a negative charge are called *anions* (−) and are attracted to the anode (+).

Beaker of water

Flashlight bulb

Battery

If we put sodium chloride (NaCl) in a beaker and raise the beaker so the electrodes are immersed in the solution,

a What will happen to demonstrate that electricity has been conducted?_____

The bulb will light.

_____

cathode

b Where will the sodium (Na^+) go? To the (cathode? anode?).

anode

c Where will the chloride (Cl^-) go? To the (cathode? anode?).

Measurement of electrolytes

34 To study body fluids, we must have suitable units of measurement. To measure volume of fluids, we use the metric system and measure in liters (L) or milliliters (ml). A milliliter is one thousandth of a liter and is generally considered the same as a cubic centimeter (cc). Therefore we may say that a liter is equal to 1000 cc. In common usage 1 cc is equal to 1 ml.

A milliliter is what fraction of a liter? ($\frac{1}{10}$? $\frac{1}{100}$? $\frac{1}{1000}$?).

$\frac{1}{1000}$

35 We must have a unit of measure for the various electrolytes in the body fluid. Since we are interested in the action of electrolytes (their ability to combine and form other compounds), the unit of measure must express

9

their combining power (chemical activity). The combining power is a function of the number of ions. The weight of the ion has no relation to the chemical activity of the ion. Measuring electrolytes in units of weight such as milligrams per 100 ml does not tell us the chemical combining power of the electrolytes in solution (i.e., how many cations, or positive ions, will be available to combine with anions, or negative ions). For example, if a hostess is having a party and wants couples of boys and girls, she does not invite 1000 pounds of boys for every 1000 pounds of girls. Their weight is not as important as the number of boys that will pair up with an equal number of girls. In measuring electrolytes, we are not concerned with how much they weigh (mg/100 ml). We want to know how many ions are available for chemical interaction. (An equal number of cations and anions is necessary.)

activity (combining power)

a We want to know the chemical _____ of the electrolytes in solution.

ions

b The chemical combining power of an electrolyte tells us how many _____ are available.

36 The unit of measure that expresses the combining activity of an electrolyte is the milliequivalent (mEq). An equivalent weight is the amount of one electrolyte that will displace or otherwise react with a given amount of hydrogen. Hydrogen is used as the yardstick or measure. One milliequivalent of any cation will always react chemically with 1 mEq of an anion, just as one boy reacts with one girl to make a couple.

100

a 100 mEq of cation will react chemically with _____ mEq of anion.

20

b 20 mEq of sodium (Na^+) will react with _____ mEq of chloride (Cl^-).

155

c If extracellular fluid has 155 mEq of cation, the number of milliequivalents of anion necessary for balance will be _____.

37 Milliequivalents provide information about the number of anions or cations available to combine with other cations or anions. For example, if the level of sodium cations in the blood is 140 mEq/L, this means that 140 cations are available to combine with 140 anions for each liter of blood. The average level of chloride ions in the blood is 104 mEq/L. Therefore, for each liter of blood, approximately 36 mEq of sodium is available to combine with some anion other than chloride.

The milliequivalent is a useful measure to compare
chemical activity _____ of electrolytes.

38 The fluid in each of the compartments (intracellular, interstitial, and intravascular) contains electrolytes. Each compartment has a particular composition of electrolytes, which differs from that of the other compartments. To function normally, body cells must have fluids and electrolytes. Furthermore, the electrolytes must be in the right compartment in the right amount. If you put lettuce out in the sun, it will become wilted. You can make the lettuce crisp by placing it in salted ice water. In the body, when potassium is lost from the cell, the person becomes weak. If the potassium is not replaced, the person will die of myocardial necrosis and circulatory failure. (The heart muscle becomes soft, dies, and cannot pump blood, since the muscle and nerve fibers are not activated because of the lack of potassium within the cell.) A specific kind and amount of certain electrolytes must be available for normal cell function.

Normal function of body cells depends on the avail-
electrolytes ability of certain _____.

39 When potassium is lost from the intracellular fluid, some other cation must replace it. Sodium, the most available cation in the extracellular fluid, moves into the cell.
equal (balanced) **a** The anions and cations must be _____.
10 **b** 10 mEq of cations will react with exactly _____ mEq of anions.

SUMMARY

Fluids and electrolytes are essential for health. The fluid compartments are the intracellular and the extracellular; the extracellular compartment includes interstitial and intravascular fluids. The body fluids contain water and electrolytes, the substances that dissociate in

11

water to electrically charged atoms called *ions*. The chemical combining power of an electrolyte is a measure of the number of ions. Electrolytes are measured in milliequivalents, which express their combining power. One milliequivalent of any cation will always react chemically with one 1 mEq of any anion. Whenever an electrolyte moves out of a cell, another electrolyte moves in to take its place. The number of cations and anions must be the same for homeostasis to exist.

REVIEW

1 The three fluid compartments in the body are

intracellular

a _____

intravascular

b _____

interstitial

c _____

substances that disso-
ciate in solution into
electrically charged
particles called ions

2 Electrolytes are _____

_____

_____

_____.

chemical combining
power

3 The number of ions available tells us the _____
_____ of an electrolyte.

the same number of

4 To achieve balance or equilibrium, we must have (more? the same number of? fewer?) anions than (as) cations.

Another cation moves in.

5 When one cation (e.g., K^+) moves out of a cell, what happens? _____

_____

NORMAL ELECTROLYTE COMPOSITION OF THE FLUID COMPARTMENTS

40 Refer to the diagrams on page 13 and answer the following questions:

a The major cation in both interstitial and intravascular

sodium

fluid is _____.

b The total milliequivalents of anion are equal to the

cation

milliequivalents of _____.

Electrolyte composition

Intravascular

Electrolyte composition of serum in intravascular compartment (mEq/L)

Cations			Anions	
H.HCO₃				H.HCO₃
Na⁺	142		104	Cl⁻
			27	HCO₃⁻
			2	HPO₄⁻⁻
			1	SO₄⁻⁻
K⁺	5		5	Organic acids
Ca⁺⁺	5		16	Protein
Mg⁺⁺	3			
Total	155		Total 155	

Interstitial

Electrolyte composition of interstitial fluid (mEq/L)

Cations			Anions	
H.HCO₃				H.HCO₃
Na⁺	145		116	Cl⁻
			27	HCO₃⁻
			3	HPO₄⁻⁻
			2	SO₄⁻⁻
K⁺	4		5	Organic acids
Ca⁺⁺	3		1	Protein
Mg⁺⁺	2			
Total	154		Total 154	

Intracellular

Electrolyte composition of intracellular fluid (mEq/L)

Cations			Anions	
K⁺	135		83	HPO₄⁻⁻
			75	Protein
			5	Cl⁻
Mg⁺⁺	42		14	SO₄⁻⁻
Na⁺	10		10	HCO₃⁻
Total	187		Total 187	

13

c The fluid compartment that has the most protein is the _____.

d The chief cation in intracellular fluid is _____.

e There is (more? similar? less?) sodium in intracellular fluid than (as) in intravascular fluid.

f The chief anion in interstitial and intravascular fluid is _____.

MOVEMENT OF FLUID IN THE BODY

41 We have considered differences in composition of the intracellular, interstitial, and intravascular fluids. These differences in composition are partially due to the nature of the barriers that separate the fluids. Cell membranes separate the interstitial fluid from the intravascular fluid. However, these barriers are selectively permeable (i.e., the cell membrane and the capillary wall will allow water and some solutes free passage through them). The *solute* is the substance that is dissolved. For international travel you must have a passport to allow entrance into another country and return to your homeland; but certain countries, such as the United States and Canada, allow free passage without a passport. Accordingly, water and some solutes freely pass through the cell membrane and the capillary wall. We shall discuss later (frame 71) some ways in which the body requires a special transport system for certain substances.

a Movement of water through the capillary wall is (unrestricted? restricted?).

b (Some? All?) solutes are allowed free passage through the walls of cells and capillaries.

42 There are several forces that affect the movement of water and solutes through the walls of cells and capillaries. We really have a mass-transportation system to carry the traffic between the fluid compartments. These forces must carry the molecules of water, foods, gases, wastes, and many kinds of ions. One process by which a solute (gas or substance) in solution moves is called *diffusion*. Diffusion is the movement of particles in all directions through a solution. When you pour a small amount of cream into a cup of black coffee, the cream mixes or spreads through the whole cup of coffee (i.e., diffuses throughout the coffee).

The process by which particles spread in all directions through a solution is called _____.

diffusion

43 Diffusion is the process by which a solute may spread throughout a solution or solvent. While a solute is the substance that is dissolved, a *solvent* is the solution in which the solute is dissolved.

solute

a A substance that is dissolved is called the (solute? solvent?).

solvent

b The solution in which a solute is dissolved is called the (solute? solvent?).

44 The particles (molecules or ions) of a substance dissolved in a solvent are moving continuously. If they are abundant in one area, they will bump into each other, causing the particles to spread from an area where there are more to an area where there are fewer particles. Thus molecules or ions diffuse from an area of high concentration to one of lower concentration.

lower

Diffusion of a solute spreads the molecules from an area of high concentration to an area of _____ concentration.

45 We have been discussing the diffusion of a solute throughout a solvent. Diffusion may also occur across a membrane if the membrane is permeable, or allows free passage. When a membrane is permeable to a certain substance, that substance can go through the membrane freely. A permeable membrane will allow substances to pass through it without restriction. However, all the membranes in the body are selectively permeable, or semipermeable.[1] A selectively permeable membrane will allow some solutes to pass through without restriction but will prevent other solutes from passing freely.

selectively

All the membranes in the body are (selectively? freely?) permeable to all substances.

46 Diffusion occurs within fluid compartments and from one compartment to another if the barrier between the compartments is permeable to the diffusing substances.

15

Diffusion is a very important process by which the solute and/or solvent may move freely from one fluid compartment to another. For example, the oxygen in the air we breathe enters the intravascular compartment and then the cells by diffusion.

One process for the movement of fluids and (some? all?) solutes is diffusion.

some

47 Now we shall consider another process, *osmosis*. If a membrane is permeable to water but not to all the solutes present, it is a selective or semipermeable membrane. When the solvent or water moves across this membrane, we call the process osmosis.

The movement of fluid through a selectively permeable membrane is called _____.

osmosis

48 Osmosis is the movement of solvent molecules across a membrane to an area where there is a higher concentration of solute that cannot pass through the membrane.

Osmosis is the movement of (solute? solvent?) across a selectively permeable membrane.

solvent

49

Before osmosis   After osmosis

1 = Dilute salt solution
2 = Concentrated salt solution
3 = Selectively permeable membrane

a Before osmosis the quantity of solution on both sides of the selectively permeable membrane is (different? the same?).

the same

b After osmosis the quantity of solution on both sides of the membrane is (different? equal?).

different

c (Solute? Solvent?) has moved.

Solvent

d The reason the solvent moved is that the membrane will not allow the solute to go through; therefore the membrane is (permeable? selectively permeable?).

selectively permeable

e After osmosis the concentration of salt solution on the two sides of the membrane is (the same? different?).

the same

16

50 All normal living membranes are selectively permeable (i.e., they do not allow all solutes free passage).

The movement of water through such membranes is

osmosis — by _____.

51 Earlier we established that particles move from an area of high concentration to an area of lower concentration. It may sound as though osmosis is the opposite. Remember, however, that a membrane is selective and allows the water to pass through but does not allow the solute through. So it is the water that is moving from an area where there is a greater amount of water in relation to solute to an area where there is less water in relation to solute.

The result of osmosis is two solutions, separated by a

equal — membrane, that are (equal? unequal?) in concentration.

52 When you have a more concentrated solution on one side of a selectively permeable membrane and a less concentrated solution on the other side, there is a pull called *osmotic pressure* that draws the water through the membrane to the more concentrated side, or the side with more solute.

Osmotic pressure is the force that draws the water from a less concentrated solution through a selectively

more — permeable membrane into a (less? equally? more?) concentrated solution.

53 The amount of osmotic pressure is determined by the relative number of particles of solute on the side of greater concentration. Therefore the greater the number of particles in the concentrated solution, the more pull there will be to move the water through the membrane.

The force that pulls water across the membrane from the side of a less concentrated solution into a more con-

osmotic pressure — centrated solution is called _____

_____.

54 When the solutions on both sides of a selectively permeable membrane have established equilibrium, or are equal in concentration, they are isotonic. *Iso-* is a combining form that means alike.

When the solutions on both sides of a selectively

permeable membrane are alike in concentration, they are

isotonic _____.

55 One of the problems in clinical medicine is the maintenance of adequate body fluids and proper chemical balance between the intracellular and the extracellular fluids. The movement of water through the cell membrane normally occurs so rapidly that any lack of osmotic balance is corrected within seconds. Therefore a state of osmotic equilibrium is maintained constantly when the body is functioning normally. When an extracellular fluid has the same concentration as the intracellular fluid, there is no net shift of fluid from outside the cell to inside the cell. The term *net* means that which remains after the deduction of all loss or gain. There is some movement of fluid, but there is no resultant change in quantity.

isotonic Therefore in this situation the extracellular fluid is like, or _____ with, the intracellular fluid.

56 An example of an isotonic solution is 0.85% sodium chloride, which is referred to as *isotonic saline* solution or *normal saline* solution. This means that it is isotonic to human cells and thus there will be very little osmosis.

0.85 An example of a solution that is isotonic to body cells is ____% sodium chloride.

57 Another example of an isotonic solution is 5% glucose.

will not be When we say a solution is isotonic to another solution or to the intracellular fluid, we mean there (will be? will not be?) movement of fluid from one side of the membrane to the other side by osmosis.

58 When a solution contains a lower concentration of salt than another solution, we say it is hypotonic. *Hypo-* means less than ordinary. A hypotonic solution has less salt, or more water, than an isotonic solution.

less A hypotonic solution has (more? less?) salt than an isotonic solution.

59 Distilled water is an example of a hypotonic solution, since it does not have solutes in it. If we put distilled water on one side of a selectively permeable membrane and normal saline solution (0.85% sodium chloride) on the other side, water will move from the distilled water side to the normal saline side to make the solutions on both sides of the membrane more nearly equal in concentration.

Distilled water is an example of (a hypotonic? an isotonic?) solution.

a hypotonic

60 We would never do this to a person, but if distilled water were injected into the bloodstream, the red blood cells would draw water into themselves. Since distilled water is hypotonic to the cells, osmosis would continue, in an attempt to bring about balance or equality, until the cells swelled and eventually burst if the situation were not changed.

A cell placed in a very hypotonic solution will (swell? shrink?).

swell

61 A solution that has a higher concentration of solutes than another solution is a hypertonic solution. We say a person who is overactive is hyperactive, *hyper-* meaning more than usual. A 10% solution of sodium chloride is an example of a hypertonic solution. A 10% solution of sodium chloride is too hypertonic to be injected into a person, but if we mix a 10% sodium chloride solution with red blood cells, water will move out of the cells and into the hypertonic solution. As the cells lose their fluid, they will become wrinkled and shriveled like prunes (i.e., crenated).

Crenated means ⸻.

wrinkled and shriveled

62 If either extreme (swelling or shriveling of the cells) occurs in a person, death will result. Fluids and electrolytes must be kept in balance for health. When they remain out of balance, death occurs. If a strong salt solution is injected into the extracellular fluid, water will be pulled out of the cells to go where the salt is.

a Shriveling happens because the salt solution is (hypotonic? hypertonic?) to the intracellular fluid.

hypertonic

b Swelling occurs if the cells are in a (hypotonic? hypertonic?) solution.

hypotonic

63 If the body loses more electrolytes than fluid, such as can happen in diarrhea, then the extracellular fluid will contain fewer electrolytes, or less solute, than the intracellular fluid.

pulled into

Therefore the fluid will be (pulled into? pushed out of?) the cells.

64 The osmotic pressure of a solution is proportional to the number of particles per unit volume of solvent. The unit of measure of osmotic pressure is the *osmole*. Therefore the ability of solutes to cause osmosis and osmotic pressure is measured in terms of osmoles. In the body the osmole is too large a unit for satisfactory use in expressing osmotic activity. The term *milliosmole* (mosm), which equals $\frac{1}{1000}$ osmole, is used to measure osmotic pressure in the body.

milliosmoles

In the body the osmotic pressure is measured in _____ (mosm).

65 Another term we will use is *osmolality*. Osmolality means the number of osmotically active particles per kilogram of water.

osmolality

The osmotic pull of all particles per kilogram of water is called _____.

66 Osmolality refers to the number of osmotically active particles per kilogram of water. A closely related term is *osmolarity*. Osmolarity refers to the number of osmoles per liter of solution.

osmolarity

The osmotic pull of all particles per liter of solution is called _____.

67 In clinical practice the difference between osmolality and osmolarity is not significant. Osmolality is measured in milliosmoles per kilogram of water (mosm/kg) and osmolarity in milliosmoles per liter (mosm/L) This difference is negligible because of the low solute concentrations in body fluids.

is not

The difference between osmolality and osmolarity (is? is not?) important in body fluids.

68 Another way to think about osmolality is as the "specific gravity" of body fluids. Since specific gravity is the weight of the solution compared with an equal volume of distilled water, the osmolality of a solution can be estimated by the specific gravity. The normal osmolality of plasma is 280 to 294 mosm/kg.

280 to 294

The normal osmolality of plasma is _____ mosm/kg.

69 The osmolality of the extracellular fluid is determined mainly by the extracellular fluid concentration of sodium. Sodium is the most abundant extracellular cation and therefore provides 90% to 95% of the effective osmotic pressure of the extracellular fluid.

The osmolality of the extracellular fluid is determined

sodium

mainly by _____.

70 Because of osmotic equilibrium, normally the extracellular fluid and the intracellular fluid have nearly the same osmolality.

280 to 294

Normal osmolality of plasma is _____ mosm/kg.

71 The processes of diffusion and osmosis are passive processes (i.e., they do not require energy from body cells). The natural tendency of molecules or ions is to move from areas of high concentration to areas of lesser concentration. In diffusion the molecules move to areas of lesser solute concentration, and in osmosis the molecules move to areas with less solvent.[5] An active transport system moves molecules or ions "uphill" against concentration and osmotic pressure. The energy for active transport is supplied by metabolic processes in the cells. Substances that are actively transported through the cell membrane include ions of sodium, potassium, calcium, iron, and hydrogen, some of the sugars, and the amino acids. An example of an active transport substance is insulin, which provides for transport of glucose from the extracellular compartment into the cell. We might liken the active transport system to a ski lift hauling skiers up a mountainside and then returning for more after dropping them at the top. Active transport systems exist for all the important electrolytes. Thus, while solutes may move by diffusion and solvents by osmosis from areas of high concentration to areas of low concentration, substances may be moved in the opposite direction by the active transport system.

When an ion moves through a membrane from an area where it is less concentrated to an area where it is more concentrated, a/an _____ system is required.

active transport

72 We have considered the movement of fluids and electrolytes in the body by diffusion, osmosis, and active transport. Another factor that influences the movement of fluids and electrolytes is *hydrostatic pressure.* Hydrostatic pressure is the force of fluid pressing outward against the vessel wall. When we relate hydrostatic pressure to the blood, we are referring not only to the pressure of the weight of the fluid against the wall of the capillary, but also to the force with which the blood is propelled by each heartbeat. Because of the force of the blood pressure, the hydrostatic pressure at the arterial end of the capillary is approximately twice as great as at the venous end.

Hydrostatic pressure is greater at the (arterial? venous?) end of the capillary.

arterial

73 When there is a difference in the hydrostatic pressure on two sides of a membrane, water and diffusible solutes move out of the solution that has the higher hydrostatic pressure. We call this process *filtration.*

The process by which water and solutes pass through a membrane when the hydrostatic pressure is greater on one side of the membrane than on the other is called _____.

filtration

74 This tells us that hydrostatic pressures cause fluid and solutes, including nutrients, to be pushed out at the arterial end of the capillary.

Hydrostatic pressure in the arterial end of the capillary results in fluid and solutes _____ _____.

leaving the capillary (being pushed out)

75 Since there is fluid in the interstitial space, there is also hydrostatic pressure in the interstitial space from the weight of the fluid. However, the hydrostatic pressure is greater inside the arterial end of the capillary (because of the heartbeat) than is the interstitial hydrostatic pressure. Therefore fluid moves out of the capillary and into the interstitial space.

Fluid moves out of the capillary at the arterial end and into the interstitial tissue because of the difference in _____ pressure.

hydrostatic

76 We established earlier that this movement of fluid and diffusible solutes (those the capillary will allow through) is called *filtration*.

Filtration is the movement of fluid through a selectively permeable membrane from an area with higher hydrostatic pressure to an area with _____ hydrostatic pressure.

lower

77 If the hydrostatic pressure at the arterial end of a capillary is 37 mm Hg and the hydrostatic pressure of the interstitial fluid is 1 mm Hg, the resultant difference, or pressure gradient, will be 36 mm Hg and fluid will be pushed out of the capillary.

Therefore fluid will move (out of? into?) the arterial end of the capillary.

out of

78 However, we must remember that osmotic pressure also affects the movement of fluid between the intravascular and interstitial compartments. Remember: osmosis is the movement of solvent molecules across a selectively permeable membrane, and osmotic pressure (or pull) is determined by the number of particles of solute on the concentrated side. The osmotic pressure due to plasma colloids, or solutes, is called the *colloid osmotic* pressure or *oncotic* pressure.

Oncotic pressure is the osmotic pressure that is due to plasma _____.

solutes or colloids

79 Turn back to page 13 and look at the difference in the protein content between the intravascular and interstitial fluid.

The larger amount of protein is in the (intravascular? interstitial?) fluid.

intravascular

80 This tells us that the oncotic pressure, or pull, will tend to move fluids (into? out of?) the capillary or intravascular compartment.

into

81 Let us look at the result of these two forces, hydrostatic pressure and oncotic pressure, when we have both of them in the same place. At the arterial end of the capillary, the hydrostatic pressure is pushing water and solutes out, whereas the oncotic pressure is pulling water in. If the blood has an oncotic pressure of 26 mm Hg and the interstitial fluid an oncotic pressure of 1 mm Hg, the oncotic pressure gradient will be 25 mm Hg. The hydrostatic pressure gradient will be 36 mm Hg, and the oncotic pressure gradient will be 25 mm Hg, resulting in an 11 mm Hg pressure difference, which will cause filtration, or movement out of the arterial capillary.

Arterial end of capillary—hydrostatic pressure

Blood hydrostatic pressure	37 mm Hg
Interstitial fluid hydrostatic pressure	− 1 mm Hg
Hydrostatic pressure gradient	36 mm Hg

Arterial end of capillary—osmotic pressure

Blood osmotic (oncotic) pressure	26 mm Hg
Interstitial fluid osmotic pressure	− 1 mm Hg
Osmotic pressure gradient	25 mm Hg

Thus

Filtration force = Hydrostatic pressure gradient	36 mm Hg
Osmotic force = Osmotic pressure gradient	−25 mm Hg
Net filtration force	11 mm Hg

greater   **a** The blood hydrostatic pressure is (greater? less?) than the interstitial fluid hydrostatc pressure.

greater   **b** The blood osmotic pressure is (greater? less?) than the interstitial fluid osmotic pressure.

greater   **c** The filtration force is (greater? less?) than the osmotic force.

out of   **d** The result is that water and solutes move (into? out of?) the capillary at the arterial end.

82 We shall now move over to the venous end of the capillary. In frame 72 we established that the hydrostatic pressure is about half as great at the venous end of the capillary as it is at the arterial end. We have the following situation at the venous end:

Venous end of capillary—hydrostatic pressure

Blood hydrostatic pressure	17 mm Hg
Interstitial fluid hydrostatic pressure	− 1 mm Hg
Hydrostatic pressure gradient	16 mm Hg

Venous end of capillary—osmotic pressure

Blood osmotic pressure	26 mm Hg
Interstitial fluid osmotic pressure	− 1 mm Hg
Osmotic pressure gradient	25 mm Hg

Thus

Osmotic force	25 mm Hg
Filtration force	− 16 mm Hg
Net osmotic pressure	9 mm Hg

less

a At the venous end the blood hydrostatic pressure is (greater? less?) than the osmotic force.

into

b The result is that at the venous end of the capillary, water and solutes move (into? out of?) the capillary.

Because of hydrostatic pressure and osmotic pressure, fluid and selected solutes move out of the capillary at the arterial end, whereas fluid and some solutes move into the capillary at the venous end.

osmotic (oncotic)

Fluids and solutes enter the capillary at the venous end because of _____ pressure.

83 About nine tenths of the fluid that filters out of the capillary at the arterial end is resorbed at the venous end. The other tenth of the fluid is returned to the vascular system by the lymph channels. The lymphatics can carry proteins and large particulate matter, which cannot be absorbed directly into the venous capillary, away from the tissue spaces. The permeability of the capillary wall varies in different parts of the body. For example, the capillaries in the liver allow protein through their membrane, whereas the capillaries in the renal glomeruli normally do not allow protein through their walls.

solutes

Capillary walls differ in permeability to (solutes? solvents?).

84 One example of a disturbance in the movement of fluids is in persons with pump failure (congestive heart failure) that goes on to pulmonary edema. In this situation the hydrostatic pressure in the lungs becomes severely increased. The hydrostatic pressure is increased so much that it overrides or exceeds the colloid osmotic pressure in the capillaries. The result is that large amounts of fluid from the capillaries move into the interstitial spaces in the lung.

a When the hydrostatc pressure in the capillaries exceeds the colloid osmotic pressure, fluid moves (into? out of?) the capillaries.

out of

b When the hydrostatic pressure exceeds the colloid osmotic pressure in the capillaries, fluid moves into the (capillaries? interstitial spaces?).

interstitial spaces

SUMMARY

Throughout the body the cell membranes and capillary walls are selectively permeable. Water and some solutes pass through the barrier freely, whereas other solutes require an active transport system.

Diffusion is the process by which a solute may spread throughout a solution. Molecules of a substance dissolved in a solvent spread by diffusion from an area of higher concentration to an area of lower concentration.

Osmosis is the movement of solvent molecules across a selectively permeable membrane to an area where there is a lesser concentration of solvent that can pass through the membrane. Since the solute cannot go through the membrane, the solvent moves to the area of lesser solvent concentration. The result of osmosis is two solutions, separated by a membrane, that are more nearly equal in concentration.

Osmotic pressure is the force that draws the solvent from a solution with more solvent activity through a selectively permeable membrane to a solution with less solvent activity. The amount of osmotic pressure is determined by the relative number of particles of solute on the side of greater concentration. When the solutions on each side of a selectively permeable membrane are equal in concentration, they are isotonic. A hypotonic solution has less solute than an isotonic solution, whereas a hypertonic solution contains more solute. If the selectively permeable membrane will allow the solvent to pass

26

through but will not allow the solute through freely, the solvent will move to the side of greater solute concentration. If an ion is to move through a membrane from an area of low concentration to an area of high concentration, an active transport system is necessary.

Osmolality refers to the number of osmotically active particles per kilogram of water. In the body osmotic pressure is measured in milliosmoles. The normal osmolality of plasma is 280 to 294 mosm/kg.

Hydrostatic pressure is the force of the fluid pressing outward against some surface. When there is a difference in the hydrostatic pressure on two sides of a membrane, water and diffusible solutes move out of the solution that has the higher hydrostatic pressure. This process is called *filtration*. At the arterial end of the capillary, the hydrostatic pressure is greater than the osmotic pressure. Therefore fluid and diffusible solutes move out of the capillary. At the venous end the osmotic pressure, or pull, is greater than the hydrostatic pressure, and fluids and some solutes move into the capillary. The excess fluid and solutes remaining in the interstitial space are returned to the intravascular compartment by the lymph channels.

REVIEW

1 The process by which particles spread in all directions through a solution is called _____.

diffusion

2 The movement of fluid through a selectively permeable membrane is called _____.

osmosis

3 The force that draws solvent from a solution with more solvent through a selectively permeable membrane into a solution with less solvent is called _____ _____.

osmotic pressure

4 When the solutions on both sides of a selectively permeable membrane are alike in concentration, they are _____.

isotonic

5 If cells are placed in a hypotonic solution, they will _____ and may _____.

swell; burst

6 The process by which water and solutes pass through a membrane when the hydrostatic pressure is greater on one side of the membrane than on the other is called

filtration _____.

7 Water and some solutes move out of the capillary at the arterial end because the hydrostatic pressure gradient

osmotic is greater than the _____ pressure gradient.

8 At the venous end water and some solutes move into the capillary because the filtration force is less than the

osmotic (oncotic) _____ force.

NORMAL MECHANISM BY WHICH WATER AND ELECTROLYTES ENTER AND LEAVE THE BODY

85 Normally water enters the body through three sources: oral liquids, water in foods, and water formed by oxidation of foods. Electrolytes are present in both foods and liquids. With a normal diet, an excess of essential electrolytes is taken in and the unused electrolytes are excreted.

Water is taken into the body through three sources. They are

oral liquids **a** _____

water in foods **b** _____

oxidation of foods **c** _____

86 The typical amount of intake for an adult is as follows:

Ingested liquids	1500 ml
Water in foods	700 ml
Water from oxidation	200 ml
TOTAL	2400 ml

The largest quantity of water is taken into the body

oral (ingested) liquids as _____.

87 Infants ingest and excrete a greater amount of fluid per kilogram of body weight than do older children or adults. An infant at age 3 months who weighs 5.4 kg requires 140 to 160 ml/kg, or 750 to 850 ml of fluid, over

Table 1. Calculation of maintenance fluids in children

Child's weight	Kilogram body weight formula
0-72 hr old	60-100 ml/kg
0-10 kg	100 ml/kg (may increase up to 150 ml if renal and cardiac function adequate)
11-20 kg	1000 ml for the first 10 kg + 50 ml for each kg over 10 kg
21-30 kg	1500 ml for the first 20 kg + 25 ml/kg for each kg over 20 kg

From Hazinski, M.F.: Nursing care of the critically ill child, St. Louis, 1984, The C.V. Mosby Co.

a 24-hour period. At age 6 months, an infant who weighs 7.3 kg requires 130 to 135 ml/kg, or 950 to 1100 ml of fluid, over a 24-hour period.[12]

more

a Infants need (more? less?) fluid per kilogram of body weight than do adults.

130

b At 6 months of age, an infant may require (100? 130? 170?) ml of fluid per kilogram of body weight over a 24-hour period.

88 While an infant requires 130 to 160 ml/kg of fluid over a 24-hour period, an adult requires approximately 30 ml of fluid per kilogram of body weight over a 24-hour period.

less than

The fluid needs of an adult are (more than? less than? the same as?) those of an infant.

89 Fluids leave the body by several routes. One way is through the skin. Water is lost through the skin of an adult by diffusion in the amount of 300 to 400 ml/day. The amount of water lost by diffusion through the skin is obligatory (i.e., it will be lost regardless of intake). We are not aware of losing water in this way through the skin; therefore it is called *insensible* perspiration.

The amount of water lost through the skin by diffu-

300 to 400 (350)

sion is about _____ ml/day.

90 Water is also lost through the skin by perspiration —a process that we are aware of. The amount of water lost by perspiration will vary depending on the temperature of the environment and of the body. The average amount of water lost by perspiration in an adult is 100 ml/day. This amount may be increased to as much as 1.5 to 3.5 L/hr.

100

The usual amount of water lost by perspiration in an adult is _____ ml/day.

91 We are unaware of losing fluid through expired air, which is saturated with water vapor. The amount of water lost from the lungs will vary with the rate and depth of respirations. The average amount of water lost from the lungs in an adult is 300 to 400 ml/day. The water lost from the lungs and through the skin by diffusion is called insensible loss because we are unaware of losing that water.

700

In an adult the total average amount of water that we say is an insensible loss would be (100? 350? 700?) ml/day.

92 Large quantities of fluid are secreted into the gastrointestinal tract, but almost all of this fluid is resorbed. The average amount of water lost in the feces of an adult is 200 ml/day—equal to the amount of water gained through the oxidation of foods.

200

The normal amount of water lost through the feces of an adult is _____ ml/day.

93 A very large volume of electrolyte-containing liquid moves into the gastrointestinal tract and then returns again to the extracellular fluid. In an adult this amount is about 8000 ml/day. Since 8000 ml is such an enormous volume, we can understand the importance of any abnormal loss of gastrointestinal secretions. Severe diarrhea will result in the loss of large quantities of fluids and electrolytes.

serious

An abnormal loss of secretions from the gastrointestinal tract is (serious? unimportant?).

94 The organs that play a major role in regulating fluid and electrolyte balance are the kidneys. More than any other organ in the body, normal kidneys can adjust the amount of water and electrolytes leaving the body. The quantity of fluid excreted by the kidneys is determined by the amount of water ingested and the amount of waste or solutes excreted. The usual quantity of urine output for an adult is approximately 1400 ml/day. However, this will vary greatly, depending on fluid intake, amount of perspiration, and several other factors.

a The major organs that regulate fluid and electrolyte balance are the _____.

b The usual quantity of urine for an adult is _____ ml/day.

kidneys
1400

95 An infant's kidneys are immature and are unable to concentrate or dilute urine. Therefore an infant requires more water and has difficulty conserving body water.

An infant requires (more? less? the same amount of?) water per kilogram of body weight than does an adult.

more

96 The amount of urine excreted in a 24-hour period depends on fluid intake, state of health, and age. The average amount of urine output for an infant at the age of 6 months is about 450 ml in 24 hours.

a At the age of 6 months, a healthy infant excretes approximately _____ ml of urine in 24 hours.

b A child excretes approximately _____ to_____ ml of urine in 24 hours.

450
500;700

97 The average total amount of water taken into the body by all three sources is 2400 ml/day in an adult. The average total amount of water leaving the body in an adult is as follows:

Skin by diffusion	350 ml
Skin by perspiration	100 ml
Lungs	350 ml
Feces	200 ml
Kidneys	1400 ml
TOTAL	2400 ml

As long as all organs are functioning normally, the body is able to maintain balance in its fluid content.

The average total output of water from all sources is _____ ml/day for an adult.

TYPES OF IMBALANCE

We shall now discuss three types of imbalance. There may be an imbalance in the volume, in the concentration, or in the composition of body fluids.

Fluid volume

98 In the diagram below, A, B, C, and D are electrolytes. Note the levels of volume.

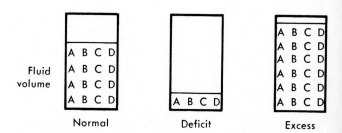

is no

a There is a deficit in volume in the middle figure of this diagram. There (is? is no?) change in the concentration or composition of the electrolytes in the fluid in this figure.

volume

b There is an excess of _____ in the third figure.

Fluid concentration

99 Besides an imbalance in the volume of fluid, another kind of imbalance is a change in the concentration of electrolytes in the fluid.

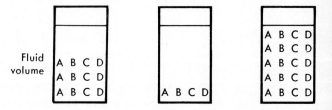

In the preceding diagram we have variations in the concentration of electrolytes in the three figures while the volume remains the same.

a The ratio of water to electrolytes in the middle figure is (increased? decreased?).

b The volume has (increased? not changed? decreased?).

c The amount of electrolyte A in each figure is (more than? equal to? less than?) the amount of electrolyte B in the same figure.

d The volume is the same in each figure. The concentration is (the same? different?).

Fluid composition

100 We shall now look at variations in composition.

```
┌─────────┐   ┌─────────┐   ┌─────────┐
│         │   │         │   │         │
│ A B C D │   │ A B C D │   │ A C C C │
│ A B C D │   │ A B C D │   │ A C C C │
│ A B C D │   │ B B C D │   │ B C C C │
│ A B C D │   │ B C C D │   │ B C C D │
│ A B C D │   │ B C D D │   │ C C C D │
└─────────┘   └─────────┘   └─────────┘
```

In each figure of the diagram the volume and the concentration of electrolytes are the same. The composition of electrolytes is different.

a In the left-hand figure the concentration of electrolytes A, B, C, and D is (equal? not equal?).

b In the middle figure there is a deficit of electrolyte _____.

c In the right-hand figure there is an excess of electrolyte _____.

SUMMARY

The electrolyte composition of extracellular fluid is different from that of intracellular fluid. Sodium is the chief cation of extracellular fluid; potassium is the major cation of intracellular fluid. At the arterial end of the capillary, hydrostatic pressure in the intravascular compartment is greater than osmotic pressure. Therefore some fluid moves out of the blood vessel. At the venous end of the capillary, fluid is drawn into the vessel because the osmotic pull is not counteracted by hydrostatic pressure. Hypertonic extracellular fluid causes the cells to shrink. Fluids cross the cell membrane by means of hydrostatic pressure and osmotic pressure. Electrolytes are transported across the cell membrane. An imbalance may occur in the volume, concentration, or composition of the fluid. If a person is to remain healthy, the fluids and electrolytes must be in balance.

REVIEW

1 The unit of measure that expresses the chemical combining power of an electrolyte is a _____.

milliequivalent

2 Fluids shift between the extracellular and the intracellular compartments by means of _____ _____ and _____.

hydrostatic pressure
osmosis

3 In the presence of a hypotonic solution, a cell will _____ and then may _____.

swell; burst

4 An imbalance in the composition of extracellular fluid means _____.

an excess or a deficit
of an electrolyte

CONTROLS FOR MAINTAINING FLUID AND ELECTROLYTE BALANCE

101 If a person is to remain healthy, the volume, concentration, and composition of fluids and electrolytes must be maintained within narrow limits. This is an extremely complex task when we consider the billions of cells in the body constantly pouring the products of chemical reactions into the extracellular fluid and withdrawing from it substances needed for specific cellular activities. What we take into the body as food and fluid contains a wide variety of materials. Some food contains electrolytes at a concentration far in excess of levels per-

missible in body fluid. The volume of liquids we drink might drown us were there no mechanisms for maintaining constant volume of body fluid. These needs for maintaining balance, or homeostasis, are multiplied in disease.

The volume, concentration, and composition of body

The volume, concentration, and composition of body fluids must be _____.

kept within limits

102 We use the term *homeostasis* to indicate the relative stability of the internal environment. The composition of the internal environment may vary from tissue to tissue because of differences in cell activity and metabolism. Yet, because of the movement of substances between the compartments, a relative constancy is maintained. We recognize, then, that the internal environment is not static but is dynamic.

Homeostasis implies (stagnation? variation within limits?).

variation within limits

103 The maintenance of homeostasis depends on a variety of processes. Substances that the cells need must be available in adequate quantity. Some of the substances required by the cell are oxygen, water, a variety of nutrients including calories, tissue-building materials, and electrolytes. The intake, storage, and elimination of the substances must be maintained within safe limits. In health the body is able to respond to disturbances in fluids and electrolytes so as to prevent or repair damage. Thirst, the conscious desire for water, is one of the major factors that determine fluid intake. The osmoreceptors in the hypothalamus are cells that are stimulated by an increase in the osmotic pressure of body fluids to initiate thirst. After eating potato chips you become thirsty because the salt on the chips increased the osmotic pressure of body fluids.

a In a healthy person one of the factors that regulate fluid intake is _____.

thirst

b When the osmotic pressure of the body fluids increases, the _____ in the hypothalamus are stimulated to initiate thirst.

osmoreceptors

104 Thirst is also stimulated by a decrease in the extracellular fluid volume. This is another way in which the

35

body attempts to regain balance—by increasing the intake of fluids.

A decrease in the volume of extracellular fluid will stimulate _____.

thirst

105 Another factor that helps to regulate water intake is dryness of the mouth due to decreased salivary secretion. However, a person who has no deficit in fluid volume will become thirsty if given atropine, a drug that prevents salivation. A dry mouth does stimulate thirst but is not necessarily limited to decreased fluid intake. In a sick person the usual stimuli may be absent or inadequate. In a healthy person, thirst is stimulated by

increased
decreased
dry

a (increased? decreased?) osmotic pressure
b (increased? decreased?) extracellular fluid volume
c (dry? moist?) mucous membranes in the mouth

106 Homeostasis of the volume of water in the body is maintained or restored by adjusting the output to the intake. The kidneys carry the major responsibility to maintain balance of both fluids and electrolytes by controlling output. They are master chemists and remove waste materials or excessive substances from the extracellular fluid. The volume of urine is regulated primarily by hormones from the posterior lobe of the pituitary gland (antidiuretic hormone) and the adrenal cortex (aldosterone). These hormones will be discussed later. Influenced by these hormones, the kidneys help to regulate the total volume of extracellular fluids, the ratio of water to solutes (concentration), and the specific quantity of the different electrolytes (composition). When the extracellular fluid volume becomes too high, the blood volume, or intravascular volume, is increased. Therefore the venous return to the heart is increased, which then increases the cardiac output. This results in an increased arterial pressure. The increased arterial pressure resulting from the increased fluid volume causes the kidneys to excrete the excess fluid.

When the volume of extracellular fluid is too high, the kidneys respond by excreting (more? less?) urine.

more

107 Normally the interstitial fluid volume is regulated so as to keep the interstitial fluid spaces filled. However, when this balance is not possible because of disease, the interstitial spaces can be expanded with excess fluid. Excess fluid in the interstitial spaces is called *edema*.

Edema is the result of increased fluid in the _____

interstitial

_____ spaces.

108 When the extracellular fluid volume is decreased because of increased loss or inadequate intake, the kidneys respond by retaining more fluid, so the extracellular fluid volume is returned to more nearly normal. However, if the extracellular fluid volume deficit is too great, the complex mechanisms affecting the kidney may not be enough to correct the imbalance, and treatment becomes necessary.

When the extracellular fluid volume is decreased, the

less

kidneys respond by excreting (more? less?) urine.

109 Two hormonal systems play major roles in regulating fluid volume. One of these is the aldosterone system. Aldosterone is a hormone secreted by the adrenal cortex that regulates the extracellular volume by affecting the renal control of sodium and potassium.

The hormone from the adrenal cortex that affects ex-

aldosterone

tracellular fluid volume is _____.

110 When the adrenal glands are overactive or the production of aldosterone is increased, sodium, chloride, and water are retained in excessive amounts. However, large amounts of potassium are excreted. Thus aldosterone affects the renal excretion or retention not only of water, but also of some electrolytes.

a When there is an increased production of aldosterone,

more

the kidneys retain (more? less?) sodium, chloride, and water.

b At the same time an increased production of aldos-

loss

terone causes a (loss? gain?) of potassium.

111 Aldosterone production is a complex and not completely understood mechanism. In a healthy person an increased production of aldosterone occurs when there is low fluid volume, low blood sodium, and high blood potassium.

Although the excretion or retention of sodium,

chloride, potassium, and water occurs through the kidneys, one of the hormones affecting this regulation is

aldosterone

_____.

112 In a healthy person the production of aldosterone is controlled to maintain a balance of fluids and electrolytes in the body. If, because of disease, the adrenal glands become overactive and secrete more aldosterone than needed for homeostasis, a serious imbalance may occur. Various diseases of the adrenal glands result in overproduction of aldosterone. Cushing's syndrome is one disease in which the adrenal glands are overactive.

You would expect the symptoms to be the result of

potassium
a excretion of _____

sodium; chloride
b retention of _____, _____,

water
and _____.

113 If the adrenal glands become extremely underactive, the excretion of potassium will be decreased or more potassium will be retained in the body. Also, the level of sodium, chloride, and water will go down because these ions are lost from the body in the urine. There are various diseases in which the adrenal glands are hypoactive.

A person whose adrenal glands are very underactive

large
will excrete a (large? normal? small?) amount of urine.

114 We have looked briefly at some ways the kidneys are influenced by the hormone aldosterone to control the volume of extracellular fluid. Another hormone that affects extracellular fluid is the antidiuretic hormone (ADH). ADH is secreted by the posterior pituitary gland. Its name explains its action, *anti-* meaning against and *-diuretic* meaning increased secretion of urine. We could say that ADH is the water-conservation hormone. It regulates the osmotic pressure of extracellular fluid by regulating the amount of water resorbed from the blood by the renal tubules.

The hormone that is secreted by the posterior pituitary

ADH (antidiuretic hormone)
gland and that acts to conserve fluid is _____.

115 The ADH mechanism is complex, but the results of the action of ADH can be summarized. If there is an

38

increased production of ADH, there will be increased amounts of water resorbed by the kidney through osmosis. The urine volume will be decreased, but the concentration will be increased.

The result of increased production of ADH is (increased? decreased?) volume of urine.

decreased

116 The usual stimulus to the production of ADH is an increase in the osmotic pressure of the extracellular fluids. ADH stimulates a retention of fluid to correct this increase in osmotic pressure. For example, if a large amount of hypertonic glucose solution is infused into the body, the osmotic pressure of the extracellular fluid will be increased. This will stimulate the production of more ADH, so more fluid will be retained and the osmotic pressure of the extracellular fluid will be returned to normal.

ADH production is regulated by changes in _____ pressure.

osmotic

117 For health to be maintained, the volume, concentration, and composition of body fluids and electrolytes must be kept within narrow limits. The regulation of these factors depends on intake and excretion.

Regulation of the loss of water and electrolytes depends primarily on the kidneys, which are affected by the hormones _____ and _____.

ADH; aldosterone

EXAMPLES OF FLUID AND ELECTROLYTE IMBALANCE

We have looked at three types of imbalance: volume, concentration, and composition. We can now talk about each separately, but we must remember that most patients will have a *combination* of imbalances.

Extracellular fluid volume imbalance

118 This type of imbalance may be a deficit in the volume of fluid without significant changes in electrolyte concentration. A deficit can be caused by an abrupt reduction in fluid intake, as when a patient is to take "nothing by mouth" (NPO). When a person is ill, there are times when neither food nor fluid is given by mouth. This may be in preparation for an anesthetic, or it may be to avoid stimulating the gastrointestinal tract. The clinical findings of fluid volume deficit include depression of the central nervous system (evidenced by reduced energy or stupor), depression of gastrointestinal activity with or without vomiting, reduced blood volume and flow of blood that leads to exhaustion, dry mucous membranes, and increased body temperature. In the treatment of extracellular fluid volume deficit without a significant change in the electrolyte concentration, fluids with electrolytes resembling the electrolytes in normal extracellular fluid are given. If the patient cannot be given fluids orally, fluids may be given parenterally (e.g., by intravenous infusion).

fluid volume

A patient who is to take nothing by mouth will have a deficit of _____.

fluids with electrolytes similar to those in normal extracellular fluid

119 In the treatment of a patient who has a deficit in fluid volume, the following are given: _____
_____
_____

Extracellular fluid concentration imbalance

120 A deficit in electrolyte concentration can occur in a patient who has a nasogastric tube in his stomach connected to suction. The patient will lose both fluids and electrolytes, especially sodium and potassium. In the treatment of this patient, fluids containing electrolytes must be given to restore the normal balance of both fluids and electrolytes. If the nasogastric tube is irrigated with water, even more electrolytes will be washed out. Therefore the tube must be irrigated only enough to keep it patent, or open. An isotonic solution such as normal saline (0.85% sodium chloride) should be used for irrigation.

sodium; potassium

A patient who has a nasogastric tube connected to suction will lose water and especially the electrolytes _____ and _____.

Imbalance in the composition of extracellular fluid

121 An example of an imbalance in the composition of electrolytes in body fluid is a deficit in potassium. A deficit in potassium can occur in infants who have diarrhea, in adults with ulcerative colitis, in burn patients who are healing, and in other conditions. Normally, when potassium (in very small quantities) moves out of the cell, sodium replaces it. This activity causes an electrochemical impulse to be transmitted along the nerve and muscle fibers. If potassium is not available in the cell, activating impulses are not transmitted to the muscles or nerves. The clinical findings include neuromuscular depression that may progress to coma. There is depression of the gastrointestinal tract with paralytic ileus (absence of peristalsis). The muscles become soft, and the electrocardiogram will show changes when the potassium deficit becomes severe and the heart cannot continue to beat.

a Activating impulses are not transmitted to the muscles or nerves when ＿＿＿＿＿＿＿＿＿＿ is not available in the cell.

potassium

b The major cation in the intracellular fluid is ＿＿＿ ＿＿＿＿＿＿＿＿＿＿.

potassium

122 When potassium has been lost from the cell because of the depletion of potassium in the extracellular fluid, several days of therapy may be needed to restore the depleted intracellular stores. Potassium may be given orally or parenterally. Remember: the exchange of fluids between the intravascular and interstitial spaces occurs rapidly through the capillary. By comparison, the rate of exchange of electrolytes across the cell membrane is slow.

If potassium is depleted in the extracellular fluid to the extent that the intracellular potassium becomes low, (minutes? hours? days?) of therapy may be required to restore the intracellular potassium level.

days

123 Since potassium is one of the ions necessary for the transmission of impulses to muscles and nerves, a severe deficit in potassium that is not corrected can be serious.

Death may result from weakness of the respiratory muscles and myocardial failure.

a deficit

Death may result from weakness of the respiratory muscles and myocardial failure when there is (a deficit? an excess?) of potassium.

SUMMARY

The volume, concentration, and composition of body fluids must remain nearly constant. The kidneys play a major role in controlling all types of balance in fluids and electrolytes. The adrenal glands, through secretion of aldosterone, also aid in controlling extracellular fluid volume by regulating the amount of sodium resorbed by the kidneys. ADH, from the pituitary gland, regulates the osmotic pressure of extracellular fluid by regulating the amount of water resorbed by the kidneys. Remember: almost any patient who has an imbalance of fluids or electrolytes will have a combination of imbalances. When one of the substances (fluids or electrolytes) is deficient, it must be replaced either normally by intake of food and water or by medical therapy—such as intravenous infusions and/or medication. When there is an excess of fluids or electrolytes, therapy is directed toward helping the body to eliminate the excess.

REVIEW

excess fluid in interstitial spaces

1 Edema is the result of _____
_____.

2 The organs primarily responsible for the regulation of volume, concentration, and composition of body fluids

kidneys

are the _____.

3 A person who has gastric suction or has had prolonged

sodium

vomiting will have a deficit of water, _____,

potassium

and _____.

4 The type of imbalance most likely to occur in a patient

a combination

is _____.

Acid-base balance/imbalance

HYDROGEN ION CONCENTRATION

124 *Acid-base balance* means homeostasis of the hydrogen ion-concentration in body fluids. Even a slight deviation in the hydrogen ion concentration causes pronounced changes in the rate of chemical reactions. Therefore survival is threatened when the hydrogen ion concentration deviates from normal. An increase in concentration of hydrogen ions (H^+) makes a solution more acidic; a decrease makes it more alkaline. The amount of ionized hydrogen in the extracellular fluid is extremely small, approximately 0.0000001 gram per liter (g/L). The number 0.0000001 may be expressed mathematically as 10^{-7}. For convenience, the minus sign is dropped and this concentration (10^{-7}) of hydrogen ions is indicated as pH 7. The symbol pH may be translated as the *power of hydrogen*; therefore the p is lowercased and the H (the symbol for hydrogen) is capitalized. Since this is a negative logarithm (exponent) of the hydrogen ion concentration, a pH of 8 would be 0.00000001 (10^{-8}), or one-tenth pH 7. Therefore the pH value falls as the hydrogen ion concentration rises; and as the concentration falls, the pH rises. (Acidity increases with a decreasing pH and decreases with an increasing pH.) The hydrogen ion concentration in body fluids determines the degree of acidity or alkalinity.

a Acid-base balance of body fluids is determined by the

hydrogen ions   concentration of _____.

b The symbol used to indicate the concentration of hydrogen ions is _____.

125 A solution is acidic, neutral, or alkaline, depending on the number of hydrogen ions present. When the number of hydrogen ions increases to a certain point, the fluid becomes acidic. We report the hydrogen ion concentration in terms of pH. *Acidity* increases as the *pH* value *decreases*.

A pH of 7.1 is more (acidic? alkaline?) than a pH of 7.6.

126 *Alkalinity* increases as the *pH* value *increases*. When hydrogen ion concentration rises, the pH value falls. Conversely, when the hydrogen ion concentration falls, the pH value increases.

A pH of 7.5 is more (acidic? alkaline?) than a pH of 7.1.

127 An acid is a substance that can give hydrogen ions, or is a hydrogen ion donor. Hydrogen ions carry a positive electrical charge and are therefore protons. Hydrogen ions are indicated by the symbol H^+.

A substance that can give up, or donate, hydrogen ions is a/an _____.

128 A substance that accepts hydrogen ions can be called a proton acceptor, or a base.

A base is a substance that (accepts? donates?) hydrogen ions.

129 Acids such as sulfuric and hydrochloric form solutions containing a high concentration of hydrogen ions when placed in water. Therefore they are regarded as strong acids. Carbonic and acetic acids are considered weak acids because in solution they provide a low concentration of hydrogen ions.

In solution a strong acid will release a (high? low?) concentration of hydrogen ions.

130 A base is a hydrogen ion (proton) acceptor. In solution a base or alkaline compound will form hydroxyl ions (OH^-).

accept

A base will (accept? give?) protons.

131 An acid will donate protons, whereas a base will accept protons. In solution a base will form hydroxyl ions (OH^-), and an acid will form hydrogen ions (H^+). One exception is ammonia (NH_3), which will accept protons to form NH_4 but will not form hydroxyl ions in solution.

a An acid will donate protons and in solution will yield

H$^+$ (hydrogen ions)

_____.

b A base will accept protons and therefore will carry a

negative

(negative? positive?) electrical charge.

132 A solution at pH 7 is neutral because at that concentration there are equal numbers of both hydrogen ions (H^+) and hydroxyl ions (OH^-), which combine to form water (H_2O). The H^+ and OH^- are completely balanced. An acidic solution has a pH value below 7; an alkaline solution has a pH value above 7. The extracellular fluid of the body is normally maintained within the range of pH 7.35 to 7.45.

alkaline

a The extracellular fluid is slightly (acidic? alkaline?).

equal (balanced)

b At pH 7 the H$^+$ and the OH$^-$ are _____.

133 The extreme limits that are compatible with life are an arterial pH of about 6.8 to 7.9. In either extreme the imbalance may result in death if not corrected.

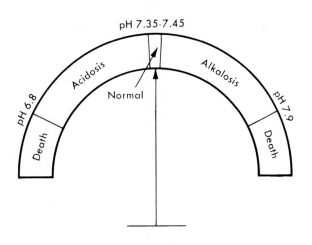

alkalosis

At a pH of 7.5 the body is in a state of _____.

134 Refer to the diagram on page 45.

a If the body fluids have a pH of 7.2, the body is in a state of _____.

acidosis

death

b If the pH goes below 6.8, _____will occur.

135 When the pH goes below 7.35, some degree of acidosis exists because there is an increase in the concentration of hydrogen ions. As the pH becomes more acidic, the central nervous system is depressed and symptoms varying from disorientation to coma result.

depress

Acidosis, an increase in hydrogen ion concentration, will (depress? stimulate?) the central nervous system.

136 When the pH goes above 7.45, some degree of alkalosis is present because there is a decrease in the concentration of hydrogen ions. Alkalosis causes an overstimulation of the central nervous system. In alkalosis the nerve cells may generate impulses even without the normal stimuli; the symptoms may range from tingling sensations in the fingers and toes to convulsions.

stimulate

Alkalosis will (depress? stimulate?) the central nervous system.

137 Slight changes in hydrogen ion concentration from the narrow range of normal pH (7.35 to 7.45) cause marked changes in the rates of chemical reactions in the cells. Some chemical reactions are depressed, and others accelerated. This is the reason why regulation of the hydrogen ion concentration is one of the most important functions of the body. The more specific effects of changes in hydrogen ion concentration will be discussed throughout the remainder of Part 2. In general, when the body is in acidosis, the patient is likely to die in coma; when the body becomes alkalotic, he may die of tetany or convulsions.

a The normal range of pH in the extracellular fluids is between _____.

7.35 and 7.45

b If the pH does not remain within these limits, the effect on cells will be one of _____ or _____chemical reactions.

increased

decreased

c Severe acidosis as well as severe alkalosis will result
in _____ if the imbalance is not corrected.

death

138 We have been considering the pH or hydrogen ion
concentration of extracellular fluid. Attempts have been
made to measure intracellular pH. However, it is impos-
sible to directly measure intracellular pH clinically for
the purpose of treating an imbalance. The intracellular
pH is generally lower than the extracellular pH, although
it varies in different organs. Intracellular pH varies in a
parallel direction with changes in the extracellular pH.
Studies indicate that the intracellular pH value of cells
may vary but is approximately 7 under normal conditions.
When the pH is measured clinically, this represents hydrogen ion concentration in the extracellular fluid.

extracellular

Clinically the (extracellular? intracellular?) fluid is
used in measuring pH.

SUMMARY

The concentration of hydrogen ions determines the
acidity or alkalinity of body fluids. The hydrogen ion concentration is indicated by pH. At pH 7 the hydrogen ions
and hydroxyl ions are balanced and the solution is neutral. The pH rises above 7 in an alkaline solution. An
acidic solution has a pH below 7. The normal pH of body
fluids is between pH 7.35 and 7.45. If the pH of body
fluids goes beyond these limits, some chemical reactions
in the body will be accelerated and others will be depressed. Either severe acidosis or alkalosis will result in
death if not corrected.

REVIEW

pH

1 The term used to indicate a measure of hydrogen ion
concentration is _____.

neutral

2 A pH of 7 is _____.

acidic

3 A pH of 7.2 is more _____ than a pH of 7.5.

47

4 A pH of 7 represents ten times the concentration of hydrogen ions as does a pH of _____.

8

5 Slight changes in the hydrogen ion concentration outside the range of normal will cause a/an _____ or _____ rate of chemical reactions in some cells.

increased
decreased

DEFENSE MECHANISMS

139 What determines the pH of extracellular fluid, and how is extracellular pH maintained? We shall discuss the pH of extracellular fluid because the pH of intracellular fluid is not measurable clinically (although intracellular pH does vary with extracellular pH). We know that the normal pH range in the body is 7.35 to 7.45. When the pH goes down, acidosis exists because there are more hydrogen ions available. In alkalosis the concentration of hydrogen ions is decreased. Normally the body maintains the pH between the narrow range of 7.35 and 7.45, even though it is constantly adding acids and bases from metabolism and from ingested food and fluids. To maintain acid-base balance, the body has three lines of defense: the buffer system, the respiratory system, and the renal system. The buffer system can act within a fraction of a second to prevent excessive changes in the hydrogen ion concentration. In 1 to 3 minutes the respiratory system working alone can readjust the concentration after a sudden change has occurred. Although the kidneys are the most powerful of the control mechanisms, if they are working alone, they will require from several hours to a day or more to readjust the hydrogen ion concentration after a sudden change. Each of the mechanisms shares the responsibility of maintaining normal hydrogen ion concentration.

The three mechanisms maintaining normal hydrogen ion concentration are

buffer system   **a** _____

respiratory system **b** _____

renal system   **c** _____

The buffer system

140 A buffer may be regarded as a chemical sponge. Depending on the circumstances, the sponge can soak up surplus hydrogen ions or release them. An acid-base buffer is a solution of two or more chemical compounds that prevents excessive changes in the hydrogen ion concentration when either an acid or a base is added to the solution. For example, if only a few drops of concentrated hydrochloric acid are added to a beaker of pure water (pH 7), the pH of the water may immediately fall as low as 1. However, if a satisfactory buffer is present, the hydrochloric acid will combine with the buffer and the pH will fall only slightly.

a The pH falls when the hydrogen ion concentration (increases? decreases?).

increases

b An acid-base buffer should prevent excessive changes in _____.

pH (hydrogen ion concentration)

141 There are a number of buffer systems in the body. However, the primary buffer system is the bicarbonate–carbonic acid system, also called the carbonate system, which consists of a mixture of carbonic acid (H_2CO_3) and sodium bicarbonate ($NaHCO_3$) in the same solution. Carbonic acid is a very weak acid; its degree of dissociation (into hydrogen ions and bicarbonate ions) is less than that of other acids. Most of the carbonic acid in solution dissociates into carbon dioxide and water, the net result being a high concentration of dissolved carbon dioxide but only a weak concentration of acid. Hydrolysis of bicarbonate in solution yields the hydroxyl ion and thus increases the alkalinity in the solution. Normally, to maintain acid-base balance (pH 7.35 to 7.45), the ratio of carbonic acid to base bicarbonate is 1:20.

$$\frac{H_2CO_3}{BHCO_3} = \frac{1}{20} = pH\ 7.4$$

There are also small amounts of potassium bicarbonate, calcium bicarbonate, and magnesium bicarbonate in the body. The symbol $BHCO_3$ is used to indicate any of these base bicarbonates.

a To maintain acid-base balance of body fluids, there

must be 1 part acid to _____ parts base in the carbonate buffer system.

b The primary buffer system in the body is the
_____ system.

carbonate

c Carbonic acid is a weak acid because most of it dissociates into _____

carbon dioxide

and _____.

water

d An increased amount of available hydroxyl ions will increase the (acidity? alkalinity?) of a solution.

alkalinity

142 When hydrochloric acid (HCl), a strong acid, is added to a solution containing sodium bicarbonate, the following reaction takes place:

$$HCl + NaHCO_3 \rightarrow H_2CO_3 + NaCl$$

Instead of the strong hydrochloric acid, we have the (strong? weak?) carbonic acid (H_2CO_3).

weak

143 Since the strong acid combines with the sodium bicarbonate to form a weak acid and sodium chloride, the hydrochloric acid that was added to the buffer solution changes the pH (slightly? excessively?).

slightly

144 When a strong acid is added in the presence of a buffer system, the pH decreases (slightly? greatly?).

slightly

145 If sodium hydroxide (NaOH), which is a strong base, is added to a buffer solution, the following reaction will occur:

$$NaOH + H_2CO_3 \rightarrow NaHCO_3 + H_2O$$

This shows that the hydroxyl ion of the sodium hydroxide combines with the hydrogen ion from the carbonic acid to form water and sodium bicarbonate.

Sodium bicarbonate is a (strong? weak?) base.

weak

146 If a strong base is added to a buffer solution, the pH will _____ only slightly.

increase

147 There are four main buffer systems in the body that help to maintain the constancy of the pH. These major buffer systems are the bicarbonate–carbonic acid system, the phosphate system, the protein system, and the hemoglobin system. Although the carbonate buffer system is not especially powerful, it is as important as the combination of all the other buffer systems in the body because *each* of the two elements of the carbonate system can be regulated through carbon dioxide content by the respiratory system and through bicarbonate ion by the kidneys. The buffer system is one of the mechanisms the body has for regulating pH.

The most important buffer in the body is the
_____ system.

The respiratory system

148 Carbon dioxide is being formed continuously in the body by the different intracellular metabolic processes. For example, the carbon in foods is oxidized to form carbon dioxide. The carbon dioxide diffuses out of the cells and into the interstitial fluids and then into the intravascular fluids. Carbon dioxide is transported to the lungs, where it diffuses into the alveoli and is exhaled. If its rate of metabolic formation is increased, its concentration in the extracellular fluids will also be increased. If the rate of pulmonary ventilation (respirations) is increased, the rate of expiration of carbon dioxide will also be increased—which will lower the amount of accumulated carbon dioxide in the extracellular fluids.

a If metabolism decreases, the carbon dioxide concentration in body fluids will (increase? decrease?).

b If the respiratory rate is decreased, the amount of carbon dioxide in the extracellular fluids will (increase? decrease?).

149 Because of the ability of the respiratory center to respond to the hydrogen ion concentration, which is the result of direct action by hydrogen ions on the respiratory center in the medulla, and because changes in respiratory ventilation in turn alter the hydrogen ion concentration in body fluids, the respiratory system acts as a feedback system for controlling hydrogen ion concentration. When the hydrogen ion concentration increases (acidosis) in the extracellular fluids, the respiratory system becomes more active (increased rate and depth of respirations) and more carbon dioxide is exhaled. Therefore the carbon dioxide concentration in the extracellular fluids decreases. Since more carbon dioxide is removed, there is less available to combine with water to form carbonic acid.

$$H_2O + CO_2 \rightleftharpoons H_2CO_3 \rightleftharpoons H^+ + HCO_3^-$$

carbon dioxide

Less carbonic acid is formed when less _____ _____ is available. Therefore the pH does not fall as it would if more carbonic acid were present in the extracellular fluid.

less

150 When the hydrogen ion concentration decreases, the respiratory system becomes (more? less?) active and the carbon dioxide concentration increases.

carbonic acid

151 If more carbon dioxide is available, more _____ _____ will be formed.

152 The respiratory mechanism for regulation of hydrogen ion concentration has an efficiency of 50% to 75%. For example, if the pH suddenly drops from 7.4 to 7, the respiratory system will return the pH to about 7.2 to 7.3 within a minute. The reason for this level of efficiency is that as the hydrogen ion concentration approaches normal, the stimulus to the respiratory center is lost. Then the chemical buffering systems, which were discussed earlier, aid in achieving balance.

partially

The respiratory system is capable of returning the pH (partially? completely?) to normal.

The renal system

153 Since the kidneys can excrete varying amounts of acid or base, they play a vital role in the control of pH. The renal regulation of body pH is a complex device for excreting varying amounts of hydrogen ions from the body, depending on the number of hydrogen ions entering the blood. This involves a series of reactions that occur in the renal tubules, including reactions for hydrogen ion secretion, sodium ion resorption, bicarbonate ion excretion into the urine, and ammonia secretion into the tubules. The bicarbonate ion entering the renal tubules changes in proportion to the extracellular bicarbonate ion concentration. When the bicarbonate ion concentration in the extracellular fluid remains normal (see the diagram on page 57), the hydrogen ion secretion and bicarbonate ion filtration normally balance and neutralize each other.

The concentration of bicarbonate ions that enter the kidneys (varies? does not vary?).

varies

154 In normal metabolism the body produces an excess of acids. To maintain balance, the kidneys excrete more hydrogen ions, and therefore the urine is usually acidic.

When more hydrogen ions are excreted in the urine, the pH of urine becomes more (acidic? alkaline?).

acidic

155 Excess hydrogen ions are excreted in the urine.

When the bicarbonate ion concentration in the extracellular fluid is greater than normal, (more? less?) bicarbonate ions than are needed to combine with hydrogen ions enter the renal tubules.

more

156 When this happens, the excess _____ _____ are excreted by the kidneys in the urine.

bicarbonate ions

157 Though the kidneys are able to excrete either an alkaline or an acidic urine, the urine is usually acidic.

When more bicarbonate ions are excreted, the urine becomes more (acidic? alkaline?).

alkaline

158 Although the renal system acts slowly, it differs from the respiratory mechanism in that it continues to act until the extracellular pH reaches exactly normal. The elderly person has a decrease in nephrons in the kidney, which may then require more time for the renal system to achieve balance. A younger adult may need 6 to 10 hours to achieve acid-base balance, whereas in the elderly person it may take 18 to 48 hours.

a The respiratory mechanism for maintaining acid-base balance has an efficiency of 50% to 75%, but the renal completely

system has the advantage of being able to neutralize (partially? completely?) the excess acid or alkali that enters body fluids.

more

b The renal system in an elderly person may require (more? same? less?) time to achieve acid-base balance than (as) that of a younger adult.

Summary of mechanisms for maintaining normal hydrogen ion concentration

The buffer system

Bicarbonate-carbonic acid (primary buffer system)	Carbonic acid (weak acid) $H_2CO_3 \rightleftharpoons H_2O + CO_2$
	Sodium bicarbonate (weak base) $NaHCO_3$
In the presence of a buffer system the pH shifts only slightly	$NaHCO_3 + HCl \rightarrow H_2CO_3 + NaCl$ (strong (weak acid) acid)
	$H_2CO_3 + NaOH \rightarrow NaHCO_3 + H_2O$ (strong (weak base) base)

The respiratory system

The respiratory system acts as a feedback system for controlling hydrogen ion concentration	H^+ concentration increases pH 7.4 → 7 Respirations →rapid and deep More CO_2 exhaled Less CO_2 to combine Therefore, less H_2CO_3
50% to 75% efficient	pH from 7 to 7.2 or 7.3 within minutes OR H^+ concentration decreases pH 7.4 → 7.8 Respirations → slow and shallow Less CO_2 exhaled More CO_2 to combine Therefore, more H_2CO_3
	pH from 7.8 to 7.6 or 7.7 within minutes

The renal system

This complex mechanism continues to act until the pH reaches normal; requires more time	Can excrete more or less H^+ to achieve balance Can excrete more or less bicarbonate to achieve balance

159 By returning some substances to body fluids and excreting others, the kidneys can compensate in several hours for even large deviations from the normal concentration of acid or base.

hydrogen ions

a If the pH of extracellular fluid goes down, the kidneys will eliminate more (hydrogen ions? bicarbonate ions?) to achieve balance.

bicarbonate

b If the extracellular fluid pH goes up, the kidneys will eliminate more (hydrogen? bicarbonate?) ions to attain balance.

SUMMARY

The homeostatic mechanisms we have considered are those that function to maintain electrolyte balance when a person is healthy. In illness the function of one of the regulating mechanisms may be affected, or the imbalance of either acid or base in the body may become too great for the body to correct without treatment.

The body has three mechanisms for the regulation of acid-base balance: the buffer system, the respiratory system, and the renal system.

The buffer system involves two or more compounds that prevent excessive changes in the pH of body fluids. The most important buffer is the bicarbonate–carbonic acid system. Carbonic acid is weak and ionizes to a limited extent.

$$H_2CO_3 \rightleftharpoons H^+ + HCO_3^-$$

Bicarbonate is a weak base and yields the hydroxyl ion.

$$HCO_3^- + H_2O \rightleftharpoons H_2CO_3 + OH^-$$

The pH of the extracellular fluid can be brought back to normal by this system.

The respiratory system helps to maintain acid-base balance through the control of carbon dioxide content. When the amount of carbon dioxide in the extracellular fluids increases, the respirations are increased in rate and depth to exhale more carbon dioxide. If the level of carbon dioxide is low, respirations are depressed. When more carbon dioxide is removed, there is less to combine with water to form carbonic acid.

The kidneys can eliminate either hydrogen ions or bicarbonate ions from body fluids and in this way can increase or decrease the pH. The renal mechanism requires more time than the other systems, but it is more powerful.

REVIEW

1 The defenses that the body has to maintain acid-base balance are

buffer system   **a** _____

respiratory system   **b** _____

renal system   **c** _____

2 The most important chemical buffer system in the body is the _____.

carbonate system

3 When a strong acid is added in the presence of a buffer system, the pH is _____.

decreased slightly

4 When the hydrogen ion concentration in the extracellular fluid increases, the respiratory system becomes _____.

more active

5 When the bicarbonate concentration in the extracellular fluids is greater than normal, the kidneys _____.

excrete more bicarbonate ions

CLINICAL CONDITIONS OF IMBALANCE

160 Any factor that decreases the rate of pulmonary ventilation will increase the concentration of dissolved carbon dioxide, carbonic acid, and hydrogen ions.

acidosis   The result of this process is (acidosis? alkalosis?).

Respiratory acidosis

161 Respiratory acidosis is caused by any clinical situation that interferes with pulmonary gas exchange and causes retention of carbon dioxide, resulting in an increase in the blood carbonic acid.

a For example, in emphysema (chronic obstructive pulmonary disease) there is obstruction to the exchange of oxygen and carbon dioxide that causes a retention of carbon dioxide, resulting in an increase of

carbonic acid

_____ in the extracellular fluid.

more

b The pH of the extracellular fluid becomes (more? less?) acid than normal.

162

a Normal balance

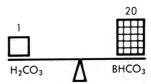

b Imbalance due to disease involving the lungs

carbonic acid

Because of disease, carbon dioxide is retained in the body; thus there is more _____ in the extracellular fluids.

hydrogen ions

c To bring about balance, the kidneys conserve base bicarbonate and excrete _____. The urine then becomes _____.

acidic

d If the body's regulating mechanisms succeed in maintaining balance, the acidosis will be compensated or corrected. If the imbalance cannot be corrected by the regulating mechanisms of the body, then medical therapy will be necessary. Treatment will be directed first at the cause (e. g., emphysema); then medication containing bicarbonate may be necessary. This usually involves solutions of sodium bicarbonate or lactate-containing solutions given intravenously. If sodium lactate is used, the lactate will be oxidized to carbonic acid, allowing the sodium to react with carbonic acid to form sodium bicarbonate. A mechanical respirator may be used to improve ventilation.

If the respiratory acidosis must be treated, the patient will need more (acid? base?).

base

163 In respiratory acidosis the problem or disease affects the respirations. Therefore the respiratory system is not available as a compensating or correcting factor.

The kidneys compensate by excreting (more? less?) hydrogen ions to return the pH to a normal level.

more

164 In respiratory acidosis the problem is excess carbonic acid that cannot be reduced by exhaling more carbon dioxide, since the respiratory system is affected by a pathological condition.

Respiratory acidosis results from an excess of _____.

carbonic acid

Respiratory alkalosis

165 In respiratory alkalosis the problem is the result of a lack of carbonic acid. Respiratory alkalosis does not occur as frequently as does respiratory acidosis.

Whenever there is excessive pulmonary ventilation of relatively normal lungs, there will be an increased loss of _____.

carbon dioxide

166 When excessive amounts of carbon dioxide are exhaled, there is a resultant (increase? decrease?) of carbonic acid in the extracellular fluid.

decrease

167 Respiratory alkalosis occurs when pulmonary ventilation is excessive and there is a decrease on the carbonic acid side of the carbonic acid-base bicarbonate ratio. Respiratory alkalosis occurs in hypoxia due to high altitude, encephalitis, or fever, because of the stimulation to the respiratory center. Salicylate poisoning, such as from an overdose of aspirin, also causes a direct stimulation of the respiratory center.

The body attempts to return the pH to normal levels through the kidneys by excreting bicarbonate ions and

retaining _____ hydrogen ions.

168

a Normal balance

b Imbalance due to disease

Respirations have increased, thus there is a loss of

carbon dioxide _____.

c To bring about balance, the kidneys excrete bicarbonate ions and retain _____.

hydrogen ions

alkaline The urine is _____.

d If the regulatory mechanism of the body cannot correct the imbalance, therapy will be directed at the cause. Included will be treatment to correct the original condition, such as the cause of a high fever. Next, carbon dioxide may be given by mask inhalation for brief intervals. Medications to increase the acid concentration will be given.

acid

In compensating for the respiratory alkalosis, both the carbonic acid and the base bicarbonate levels are decreased. Treatment is aimed at increasing the (acid? base?) side.

169 In respiratory alkalosis some factor has affected the respiratory system so that increased amounts of carbon dioxide are _____.

exhaled

bicarbonate ions

a To compensate, the kidneys excrete _____
_____.

carbon dioxide

b In the treatment _____ may be given by mask inhalation for short intervals.

Metabolic acidosis

170 Some clinical conditions that may lead to metabolic acidosis are severe diarrhea, vomiting, uremic acidosis, and diabetes mellitus. For example, in diabetes the lack of insulin prevents the use of glucose for metabolism. The stored fats are oxidized into acids. Acetoacetic acid is one of those acids and is metabolized for energy. The acetoacetic acid concentration in the extracellular fluids often rises to a very high level, and large quantities are excreted in the urine. Metabolic acidosis occurs because of the high acid content in extracellular fluid and also because the acetoacetic acid carries large quantities of sodium as sodium bicarbonate with it into the urine.

sodium bicarbonate

Metabolic acidosis results because of the high acid content of the blood, which also causes a loss of _____
_____, the alkaline half of the carbonate buffer system.

171
a Normal balance

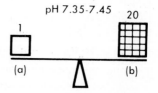

In the diagram on page 60, the labels should read

In the diagram on page 60, the labels should read

H₂CO₃, BHCP₃ (a) _____ (b) _____

b Diabetic acidosis (acetoacetic acid combines with bicarbonate)

c Regulatory mechanisms

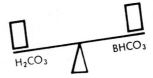

hyperactive (deep and rapid)

carbon dioxide

acidic

(1) Breathing becomes _____ (Kussmaul breathing).

(2) The lungs exhale more _____.

(3) The kidneys excrete hydrogen ions, and the urine becomes _____.

d In metabolic acidosis there is usually an extracellular fluid volume deficit that must be corrected by parenteral fluids. To treat diabetic acidosis, carbohydrates and insulin must be supplied. Intravenous solutions of sodium bicarbonate or lactate (such as sodium lactate) may also be needed to support the base bicarbonate.

base bicarbonate

Treatment is aimed at correcting the cause of the metabolic acidosis and replacing the _____ _____ deficit.

172 In metabolic acidosis there is a deficit in available

base (alkali)

_____.

a The homeostatic mechanisms that function to return the pH to a normal level include _____

respiratory, renal, and buffer systems

_____.

hydrogen ions

b The kidneys excrete _____.

7.35 to 7.45

173 The normal pH of the extracellular fluids is _____ _____.

174 In diabetic acidosis the respirations are called *Kussmaul breathing*. Since the respiratory system functions to return the pH to a more nearly normal level, the respirations become _____.

hyperactive
(deep and rapid)

Metabolic alkalosis

175 Metabolic alkalosis may be caused by ingestion of large amounts of sodium bicarbonate or by the loss of chloride through vomiting or gastric suction. When chloride is lost, the sodium that is left forms excessive sodium bicarbonate.

a Normal balance

7.35 to 7.45

    (1) Normal pH is _____.

Ratio of acid?	Ratio of base?

1:20

H₂CO₃

BHCO₃

increased

    (2) In the carbonate buffer system the ratio of acid to base is _____.

    (3) The symbol for carbonic acid is _____ ; the symbol for base bicarbonate is _____.

b Base bicarbonate is (increased? decreased?).

c Regulatory mechanisms

slow; shallow

retain

hydrogen ions

alkaline

(1) Breathing becomes _____ and _____, the lungs _____ carbon dioxide.

(2) The kidneys retain _____, causing the urine to become more _____.

d If the body's regulatory mechanisms cannot bring about balance, a chloride-containing solution will be given. The chloride ions of the solution promote excretion of the bicarbonate ions and help to relieve the base bicarbonate excess.

The major factor causing an imbalance in metabolic alkalosis is _____ excess.

base bicarbonate

176 The lungs help to return the pH to normal by _____.

conserving
carbon dioxide

Table 2. Summary of acid-base imbalance

Type	Etiology	Compensation
Respiratory acidosis (carbonic acid excess)	Chronic lung disease Surgery	Buffer system Renal system: excrete more H^+
Respiratory alkalosis (carbonic acid deficit)	Increased pulmonary ventilation Encephalitis Hypoxia Fever Salicylate poisoning	Buffer system Renal system: excrete more HCO_3^-
Metabolic acidosis (base deficit)	Diabetic ketoacidosis Uremic acidosis Diarrhea	Buffer system Respiratory system: rapid and deep Renal system: excrete more H^+, retain more HCO_3^-
Metabolic alkalosis (base excess)	Excessive ingestion of base (antacids) Vomiting Gastric suction	Buffer system Respiratory system: slow and shallow Renal system: retain more H^+, excrete more HCO_3^-

Combination of types of imbalance

177 We have considered respiratory acidosis and alkalosis and metabolic acidosis and alkalosis as separate entities. It is possible to have a combination of types of imbalance. For example, salicylates can cause two types of acid-base disturbance. First, the salicylates stimulate the respiratory center, which produces marked hyperventilation and respiratory alkalosis. The salicylates then cause a disturbance in metabolism, which results in increased accumulation of acids in the body and metabolic acidosis. When there is a combination of types of imbalance, treatment must be vigorous to prevent death.

combination

It is possible to have a single type of acid-base imbalance or a _____ of types of imbalance.

Effects of acidosis and alkalosis on the body

178 The major effect of acidosis is depression of the central nervous system. When the pH of the blood falls below 7, the nervous system becomes so depressed that the person is disoriented and later may be comatose. The main effect of alkalosis on the body is overexcitability of the nervous system. This occurs both in the central nervous system and in the peripheral nerves, with the peripheral nerves usually affected first. As a result of repeated stimulation by nerves, the muscles go into a state of tetany or tonic spasm. A patient with alkalosis may die from tetany of the respiratory muscles. The symptoms of central nervous system stimulation are nervousness and convulsions.

depression

a Acidosis causes _____ of the central nervous system.

stimulation

b Alkalosis causes _____ of the central and the peripheral nervous systems.

SUMMARY

Respiratory acidosis or alkalosis is the result of some disease or conditon that affects the respiratory system. In respiratory acidosis there is interference, causing increased amounts of carbon dioxide to remain in the body. This results in an increase of carbonic acid. In respiratory alkalosis there are decreased amounts of carbon dioxide in the body and consequently less carbonic acid. In respiratory acidosis the kidneys assume responsibility for correcting the imbalance by conserving base bicarbonate and excreting hydrogen ions. In respiratory alkalosis the kidneys excrete bicarbonate ions and retain hydrogen ions.

Metabolic acidosis is the result of a loss of base, and metabolic alkalosis results from an excessive intake of base. Therefore both the respiratory system and the renal system contribute to return the pH to the normal body level. In metabolic acidosis there are increased quantities of acid in relation to the available base in the intravascular fluid. Therefore the body compensates by hyperactive breathing to exhale more carbon dioxide, and the kidneys excrete more hydrogen ions. In metabolic alkalosis there is an increase of base in the intracellular fluid. Respirations become suppressed to increase the carbon dioxide and consequently the carbonic acid. The kidneys retain hydrogen ions and excrete bicarbonate ions to return the pH of the extracellular fluids to a normal level.

REVIEW

1 When carbon dioxide is retained in the intravascular fluid, the result is an increase of _____.

carbonic acid

2 An increase of carbonic acid in the intravascular fluid results in _____.

acidosis

3 When acidosis exists, the kidneys excrete _____ _____.

hydrogen ions

4 In metabolic alkalosis more base bicarbonate is available; therefore the respiratory system becomes _____ _____ and retains _____.

suppressed
carbon dioxide

5 In metabolic alkalosis the kidneys excrete _____ _____ and retain _____.

bicarbonate ions
hydrogen ions

6 The major effect of acidosis on the nervous system is _____.

depression

Blood gas analysis

179 In acid or base imbalance some of the effects are not very specific. Therefore the blood gas analysis is the most useful way to identify the imbalance.

The most useful test to identify an acid or base imbalance is the _____ analysis.

blood gas

180 Arterial blood is best for blood gas analysis. Arterial blood gas analysis measures pH, arterial oxygen tension (Po_2), arterial carbon dioxide tension (Pco_2), and either standard plasma bicarbonate (HCO_3^-) or carbon dioxide content. (When a gas such as carbon dioxide is dissolved in a liquid, the concentration of the gas in the liquid is directly proportional to the partial pressure. "P" stands for partial pressure.) The normal range of arterial pH is 7.35 to 7.45; the normal range of arterial Po_2 is 80 to 110 mm Hg; and the normal range of arterial Pco_2 is 35 to 46 mm Hg.

7.35 to 7.45
a The normal arterial pH is _____.

80 to 110
b The normal arterial Po_2 is _____.

35 to 46
c The normal arterial Pco_2 is _____.

181 The arterial blood gases have the same normal values in children as in adults. However, during the first month of life infants have values that are slightly lower than those of children and adults. In a newborn the pH has a normal range of 7.27 to 7.42; the normal range of arterial Po_2 is 60 to 80 mm Hg; and the normal range of Pco_2 is 30 to 40 mm Hg.

In a newborn the arterial blood gas values are (the same as? lower than? higher than?) those in a child or an adult.

lower than

182 The base component is evaluated in some laboratories by the standard bicarbonate, but in others the carbon dioxide content is used instead. The latter is a more useful test, since it measures both elements of the acid-base proportion and permits an accurate assessment of the clinical problem. The carbon dioxide content represents the sum of all forms of carbon dioxide in the blood, which includes that dissolved in the plasma (measured as P_{CO_2}), that derived from bicarbonate (HCO_3), and that derived from plasma carbonic acid (H_2CO_3). The normal carbon dioxide content is 24 to 33 mEq/L, or an average of 28 mEq/L in an adult. The normal value for standard plasma bicarbonate is 22 to 26 mEq/L in an adult.

In an infant the normal carbon dioxide content is 20 to 28 mEq/L, which is lower than that in an older child or an adult. The normal value for standard plasma bicarbonate is 22 to 26 mEq/L in an adult and slightly lower, 20 to 26 mEq/L, in an infant.

a The base component is measured by the standard bicarbonate or the carbon dioxide content. The normal average carbon dioxide content for an adult is _____ mEq/L.

b The base component, whether measured by the standard bicarbonate or the carbon dioxide content, in an infant is (slightly higher than? the same as? slightly lower than?) that in an adult.

183 In examining arterial blood gas values you should look at the pH first. The pH is the prime indicator of acidosis or alkalosis.

a A pH of 7.24 would indicate (acidosis? alkalosis?).

b A pH of 7.56 would indicate (acidosis? alkalosis?).

184 You should look at the P_{CO_2} to determine the respiratory parameter. If the P_{CO_2} is increased, it indicates that more carbon dioxide is being retained. If the P_{CO_2} is decreased, it indicates that more carbon dioxide is being exhaled. A high P_{CO_2} is an indication of respiratory acidosis.

In respiratory acidosis the P_{CO_2} will be (above? below?) normal.

185 The next part of the arterial blood gas analysis, which will help you determine the type of acid-base imbalance, is the base component. This is the metabolic parameter. The carbon dioxide content (base) will be increased in metabolic alkalosis.

In metabolic acidosis the carbon dioxide content (base) will be (increased? decreased?).

Respiratory acidosis

186 Respiratory acidosis is the result of an increased level of carbonic acid in the extracellular fluid that is caused by an inadequate exchange of gases in the lungs, with retention of carbon dioxide. Conditions that may cause respiratory acidosis include depression of respirations by drugs or disease, foreign objects in the airway, and trapping of air in portions of the lung (as occurs with emphysema and pneumonia).

Any condition in which there is retention of carbon dioxide may cause _____.

respiratory acidosis

187 Signs we need to recognize that may indicate respiratory acidosis include distressed respirations, anxiety, disorientation, confusion, and body weakness.

a One sign of respiratory acidosis is (easy? distressed?) respirations.

distressed

b A person who has respiratory acidosis is likely to be (oriented? disoriented?).

disoriented

188 If the respiratory acidosis is severe, the person may become unconscious or may develop ventricular fibrillation.

It is possible for a person in severe respiratory acidosis to develop an arrhythmia of the heart such as _____.

ventricular fibrillation

189 According to laboratory findings, in respiratory acidosis that is uncompensated the pH will be low and the partial pressure of carbon dioxide (P_{CO_2}) will be high. The carbonic acid concentration cannot be measured directly in the hospital laboratory. However, the carbonic acid concentration is proportional to the partial pressure of the carbon dioxide, and this can be measured. Since carbon dioxide is retained, the P_{CO_2} will be high. The normal range of P_{CO_2} is 35 to 46 mm Hg. The average P_{CO_2} in arterial blood is 40 mm Hg, whereas the average P_{CO_2} in venous blood is 46 mm Hg.

a The normal range for pH in extracellular fluid is

7.35 to 7.45

_____.

35 to 46

b The normal range of P_{CO_2} is from _____ mm Hg.

low

c In respiratory acidosis the pH will be (high? low?).

high

d The P_{CO_2} will be (high? low?).

190 As the buffer systems and kidneys compensate for the acidosis, the pH will return to normal. The P_{CO_2} may return to more nearly normal but likely will remain elevated if the cause of the respiratory acidosis is not corrected. The pH can return to normal even though carbon dioxide is retained in the body because the kidneys conserve bicarbonate ions and excrete hydrogen ions to achieve balance.

As the body compensates for the acidosis, the pH will

return to normal

likely (remain low? return to normal? remain high?).

191 Normal breathing must be restored as much as possible. Treatment is aimed at the cause of the inadequate exhalation of carbon dioxide. Drugs that further depress respiration should not be given.

Deep respirations at regular intervals will aid in re-

breathing

storing normal _____.

192 The elevated P_{CO_2} must be reduced gradually. Intermittent mechanical ventilation is sometimes used to help reduce the P_{CO_2}.

Mechanical ventilation may be used in treating re-

P_{CO_2}

spiratory acidosis to reduce the elevated _____.

193 The basic treatment includes maintaining a patent airway, aspiration of excessive respiratory secretions, and artificial respiration if necessary. Medications and parenteral fluids may be necessary to restore balance. In extreme cases parenteral fluids that contain lactate or bicarbonate could be used.

Adequate ventilation is the main treatment for

respiratory acidosis _____.

194 Oxygen may be used when anoxia is present. However, in a person with chronic retention of carbon dioxide · (e.g., as occurs in emphysema), oxygen may endanger the patient. Normally, as the level of carbon dioxide increases, the medulla and chemoreceptors stimulate respirations. In a person with a chronic elevation of carbon dioxide, the respiratory center becomes insensitive to the level of carbon dioxide. Respirations are stimulated instead by a decreased oxygen level.

increased **a** Normally respirations are stimulated by (increased? decreased?) carbon dioxide.

b In a person with chronic retention of carbon dioxide,
oxygen respirations are stimulated by low levels of _____.

195 If oxygen is administered to a person with a chronically elevated P_{CO_2}, observe the patient closely because respirations could be depressed to the point of cessation.

Oxygen should be used cautiously in the person with
P_{CO_2} chronic elevation of _____.

Respiratory alkalosis

196 Respiratory alkalosis results from a deficit in carbonic acid that is caused by hyperventilation. It is a common type of acid-base imbalance. Respiratory alkalosis may result from intracranial lesions or high temperature.

Any condition in which there is a loss of carbon diox-
respiratory alkalosis ide can cause _____.

197 One of the earliest signs of respiratory alkalosis is a tingling sensation in the fingers and toes. This is due to the stimulation of the nervous system. Other symptoms that may occur if the alkalosis is severe include palpitation, perspiration, tetany, and heart arrhythmias.

The earliest sign of respiratory alkalosis is a _____
tingling sensation _____ in the fingers and toes.

198 In respiratory alkalosis the laboratory findings show the pH to be higher than normal and the P_{CO_2} to be low. This is just the reverse of the laboratory findings in respiratory acidosis.

high

a In respiratory alkalosis the pH will be _____.

low

b In respiratory alkalosis the P_{CO_2} will be _____.

199 As the body compensates for the alkalosis, the kidneys will conserve hydrogen ions.

If the kidneys retain more hydrogen ions, they will

bicarbonate

excrete more _____ ions.

200 The treatment of respiratory alkalosis is aimed at increasing the level of carbon dioxide. This can be done by having the patient rebreathe a mixture of his own carbon dioxide and oxygen from a large paper bag or by giving inhalations of 5% carbon dioxide at intervals.

Treatment of respiratory alkalosis should increase the

carbon dioxide

level of _____.

Metabolic acidosis

201 A patient with mild metabolic acidosis may have no symptoms. The acidosis is due to a decrease in the alkali reserve. It may be caused by a loss of bicarbonate from the gastrointestinal tract or the kidneys or from excessive production of acid. The early symptoms include general malaise or weakness and a dull headache. Nausea, vomiting, and abdominal pain may also be present.

Early signs of metabolic acidosis include general malaise and headache that may be accompanied by the following gastrointestinal symptoms:

nausea

a _____

vomiting

b _____

abdominal pain

c _____

202 As the acidosis increases in severity, the person may become confused and finally unconscious.

In acidosis the central nervous system is depressed.

confusion; unconsciousness

Therefore _____ and then _____ may occur.

203 The laboratory findings include a low pH and a low standard bicarbonate. The normal value for standard plasma bicarbonate ranges between 22 and 26 mEq/L. Normal carbon dioxide content is 24 to 33 mEq/L, or an average of 28 mEq/L.

below

a In metabolic acidosis the pH is (above? below?) normal.

below

b If the standard bicarbonate is measured in metabolic acidosis, it will be (above? below?) normal.

content

c Instead of measuring standard bicarbonate, the laboratory may report the carbon dioxide _____.

28

d The average normal value for carbon dioxide content is _____ mEq/L.

204 A decreased pH will stimulate the respiratory center to exhale more carbon dioxide and thus reduce the carbonic acid. Therefore another symptom in metabolic acidosis is deep and rapid respirations. The laboratory values will be different in uncompensated and compensated metabolic acidosis. In uncompensated metabolic acidosis the pH will be low, the P_{CO_2} will be normal, and the carbon dioxide content will be low (as is the standard bicarbonate).

In uncompensated metabolic acidosis the standard bicarbonate will be low and the carbon dioxide content will

low

be (high? low?).

205 When compensation occurs, the pH rises slightly but may remain below normal. The P_{CO_2} falls because of hyperventilation. If the kidneys can conserve bicarbonate ions, the standard bicarbonate will rise toward normal (as will the carbon dioxide content).

In partially compensated metabolic acidosis the pH, standard bicarbonate, and carbon dioxide content will return to more nearly normal but will remain slightly

below

(below? above?) normal.

206 Treatment is aimed at correcting the cause of the metabolic acidosis. In severe acidosis fluids must be given to correct the base bicarbonate deficit. Alkalinizing solutions such as sodium bicarbonate or lactate-containing solutions may be given parenterally.

Treatment with parenteral fluids include solutions to correct the deficit of _____.

base bicarbonate

Metabolic alkalosis

207 Metabolic alkalosis is the result of excessive base bicarbonate and may occur because excessive base was taken orally or given parenterally. It also may occur when hydrochloric acid is lost from the body by vomiting or through suction.

Remember: the effect of alkalosis on the central nervous system is _____.

stimulation

208 Therefore the symptoms we can expect because of central nervous system stimulation include paresthesias (abnormal sensations such as numbness and prickling), restlessness, confusion, and tetany.

In the laboratory findings we would expect the pH to be (above? below?) normal.

above

209 The standard bicarbonate content and carbon dioxide content in metabolic alkalosis are the opposite of those found in metabolic acidosis.

In metabolic alkalosis the standard bicarbonate and carbon dioxide content will be (above? below?) normal.

above

210 The aim of treatment is to correct the problem that produced the metabolic alkalosis. Then treatment is directed at replacing lost acid in the form of fluid or medication containing chloride. In metabolic alkalosis caused by vomiting, usually there will also be a deficiency of potassium, in which case potassium chloride can sometimes be used in treatment.

A chloride-containing solution or medication would likely be used in treating _____.

metabolic alkalosis

General nursing responsibilities

211 We have considered the signs, laboratory results, and treatment for the four types of acid-base imbalance. It should be evident that overtreating one type of imbalance may upset the balance in the opposite direction. We shall now consider general nursing responsibilites in acid-base imbalance. The nurse must make pertinent observations. These will include the state of consciousness, restlessness, type of respirations, skin color, and vital signs. In observing the patient's state of consciousness, the nurse will need to know whether he is oriented, alert, or drowsy but rouses easily or whether he responds only to pain.

consciousness

The nurse must assess the state of _____ of the patient.

212 In addition to the patient's state of consciousness, the nurse should observe whether the patient is quiet or restless and the character of his respirations.

The nurse must observe whether the patient is restless and what is characteristic of the patient's

respirations

_____.

213 So far we have considered observation for state of consciousness, restlessness, and character of respirations. The nurse should also observe the skin for color changes and whether it is moist or dry.

In observing the skin, the nurse looks for changes in

color

_____ and determines whether the skin is moist or dry.

214 The nurse should observe the state of consciousness, restlessness, type of respirations, skin color and moisture, and vital signs. In taking the pulse rate, the nurse should look especially for irregularities in rhythm.

In taking the pulse, the nurse should be alert to

irregularities

_____ in rhythm.

215 In addition to making pertinent observations, the nurse must protect the patient from injury. Since a person with acid-base imbalance may have either depression or stimulation of the central nervous system, the nurse must protect such a patient from injury during unconsciousness or convulsions. Protecton of the patient from injury is an important nursing responsibility.

a In acidosis the patient will have depression of the central nervous system that could cause _____.

unconsciousness

convulsions

b In alkalosis the nervous system is stimulated, and the patient may have _____.

216 The nurse should make pertinent observations, protect the patient from injury, and provide both physiological and psychological comfort.

comfort

The nurse should provide physiological and psychological _____.

217 Another important nursing responsibility for patients with acid-base imbalance is accurate recording of intake and output. The type and volume of fluids taken as well as lost will be important in determining treatment. A record of intake and output is especially important in infants and elderly persons.

intake

output

An accurate record of both _____ and _____ is important for the patient with either acid or base imbalance.

218 The nurse should make pertinent observations, protect the patient from injury, provide comfort, and record intake and output. The nurse must also be able to perform the necessary therapeutic procedures as indicated. This might include catheterization and hourly analysis, venipuncture for diagnostic tests and parenteral fluids, and other nursing procedures.

The nurse may need to perform therapeutic procedures, such as catheterization, for the purpose of

hourly analysis

_____.

SUMMARY

Acid-base imbalance caused by a disturbance in the level of carbonic acid is called *respiratory* acidosis or alkalosis. The laboratory criteria useful in determining the degree of imbalance are the pH and P_{CO_2}. In respiratory acidosis the pH will be low and the P_{CO_2} will be high. Treatment is aimed at relieving the cause of retention of carbon dioxide and then giving base or alkali to restore balance. In respiratory alkalosis the pH will be high and the P_{CO_2} will be low. Treatment is aimed at increasing the retention of carbon dioxide.

In *metabolic* acidosis and alkalosis the problem is the level of base bicarbonate or alkali. In metabolic acidosis the level of base bicarbonate is less than normal and therefore the acid side of the balance is high. The laboratory findings include a low pH and standard bicarbonate and carbon dioxide content. Treatment is aimed at correcting the cause of the imbalance and replacing base. In metabolic alkalosis there is an excess of base, which is indicated by a high pH and standard bicarbonate and carbon dioxide content. Treatment is directed toward supplying acid.

In both types of acidosis, respiratory and metabolic, the central nervous system is depressed. The nurse must be alert for symptoms such as disorientation, confusion, lethargy, and malaise. If the degree of acidosis increases in severity, the patient may become unconscious. In respiratory acidosis respirations may be distressed. In metabolic acidosis there may be gastrointestinal symptoms of nausea, vomiting, and abdominal pain.

In both types of alkalosis, the central nervous system is stimulated. Therefore the nurse should be alert to signs of paresthesia, restlessness, confusion, and tetany. If the degree of alkalosis increases in severity, convulsions may occur.

The nurse must observe and report signs and symptoms that may indicate an acid or base imbalance. The patient must be protected from injury. The nurse should also provide comfort and keep a record of intake and output.

REVIEW

1 Distressed respirations are likely to occur in and may produce _____.

respiratory acidosis

2 A patient who has respiratory acidosis is likely to be (oriented? disoriented?).

disoriented

3 In a patient with chronic retention of carbon dioxide, respirations will be stimulated by low levels of _____.

oxygen

4 In respiratory alkalosis the P_{CO_2} will be _____.

5 Nausea, vomiting, and abdominal pain sometmes occur in _____.

6 In uncompensated metabolic acidosis the standard bicarbonate and carbon dioxide content are _____.

7 The nurse should make pertinent observations, protect the patient from injury, provide comfort, perform therapeutic procedures, and record _____ and _____.

CASE STUDIES

Jamie Smith

1 Jamie Smith is 6 weeks old, and his mother reports that he has begun to vomit after each feeding. She is breast-feeding him, and he nurses hungrily. Earlier he would occasionally "spit up" some after a feeding, but not like he has in the past few days. This morning it was projectile. Yet Jamie seems to be hungry. The vomitus smells sour and is the color of milk. You notice that his respirations are shallow and are slower than expected.

His blood gas report is as follows:

pH is 7.49

P_{O_2} is 88 mm Hg

P_{CO_2} is 35 mm Hg

CO_2 content is 37 mEq/L

a Jamie's pH of 7.49 tells you he has (acidosis? alkalosis?).

b His P_{CO_2} of 35 is _____.

c His CO_2 content of 37 is _____.

d It is likely that Jamie has _____.

2 In children the most common cause of metabolic alkalosis is loss of hydrochloric acid (HCl) through vomiting secondary to hypertrophic phyloric stenosis.

Jamie has developed metabolic alkalosis because of loss of _____.

3 It is important for Jamie to have his alkalosis corrected

77

before he has treatment for his hypertrophic pyloric stenosis. He needs to have the chloride replaced, as well as other electrolytes that may be low. It is also likely that he needs to have fluid volume replaced.

Jamie should have treatment for his metabolic alkalosis (before? after?) treatment for his hypertrophic pyloric stenosis.

before

Laura Hart

1 Laura Hart, 18 years old, has come to the physician's office with symptoms of polyuria (frequent urination), polydipsia (excessive thirst), tiredness, and muscular weakness. She is breathing deeply and rapidly.

Her laboratory findings include glucose and acetone in her urine and a blood sugar level of 560 mg/100 ml. Her plasma pH is 7.02; her Pco_2 is 19 mm Hg.; and her CO_2 content is 5 mEq/L.

acidosis

a Ms. Hart's pH of 7.02 indicates that she has (acidosis? alkalosis?).

low

b Her Pco_2 of 19 is (low? normal? high?).

very low

c Her CO_2 content of 5 is (very low? slightly low? normal? high?).

2 With her deep and rapid respirations, Ms. Hart will

carbon dioxide

lose more _____.

carbonic acid

Her rapid respirations are a defense mechanism to get rid of more CO_2 so there will be less (carbonic acid? bicarbonate?).

3 Since Ms. Hart's respiratory system can assist in compensating for her acidosis, her pH is not as low as it would

metabolic

be without that mechanism. Her acidosis is (metabolic? respiratory?).

4 Ms. Hart's treatment needs to be aimed at lowering her blood sugar level, along with adding fluids to correct the base bicarbonate deficit. Since her base bicarbonate level is lower than normal, the acid side of the balance

high

is (high? low?).

Robert Jones

1 Robert Jones is a 50-year-old man who has been admitted to the hospital in a state of coma. The history indicates that he has had chronic obstructive lung disease for the past 6 years, and during the past 2 weeks he became increasingly weak and disoriented.

Mr. Jones' blood gas report is as follows:

pH is 6.8

Po_2 is 55 mm Hg

Pco_2 is 95 mm Hg

CO_2 content is 35 mEq/L

acidosis

very high

respiratory acidosis

a Mr. Jones' pH of 6.8 tells you he has _____.

b His Pco_2 of 95 is (low? normal? high? very high?).

c Mr. Jones has _____.

2 Mr. Jones' pH of 6.8 is at the lower limit that is compatible with life. Unless he has active treatment, his acidosis will result in _____.

death

3 Mr. Jones also has hypoxia, with a Po_2 of 55, which needs to be treated along with his respiratory acidosis. Mr. Jones has a (serious? slight?) acid-base imbalance.

serious

Mary Baker

1 Mary Baker, age 8, has been practicing for this swimming race for several weeks. She is a strong swimmer, but she is afraid she will not win this one. As she is getting ready to begin the race, she is breathing rapidly and deeply so she can go as far as possible under water. Suddenly she sits down and says her lips and hands are numb. You notice that her hands are in carpal spasm. She says she feels as though she will faint.

carbon dioxide

a You know that with deep and rapid breathing, more _____ is exhaled and lost from the body.

carbonic acid

b With less carbon dioxide available, there will be a deficit of _____.

respiratory alkalosis

c The acid-base imbalance Mary has is _____.

2 The treatment for respiratory alkalosis is to increase the level of carbon dioxide. One way you could do this would be to have Mary rebreathe _____

her carbon dioxide and oxygen mixture

_____ by holding a paper bag over her mouth and nose.

Fluid volume imbalance

INTRODUCTION

Illness is usually accompanied by some disturbance of body fluids, either locally or systemically. The nurse must know what the various body fluid disturbances are, how they develop, and what characterizes them. You have completed the program that presents the normal distribution and constituents of body fluids, as well as the controls for maintaining fluid and electrolyte balance. As a nurse you share with the physician the responsibility for making observations that will serve as a basis for decisions regarding the fluid and electrolyte status of the patient. The nurse is available to make observations not only of the patient's output, but also of his intake, as well as symptoms and signs relative to his fluid needs.

Fluid volume imbalance is more likely to occur and to be severe in infants and in the elderly than in children or younger adults. The greater needs of infants for fluid and their larger surface area relative to their size contribute to their potential for fluid imbalance. In addition, infants have a higher metabolic rate with greater heat production and insensible fluid loss, along with a greater need for fluid excretion. Kidney function is immature at birth, with a limited capacity to concentrate or dilute urine. In the elderly there is homeostatic fragility along with decreased total body water. With increasing age there is a reduced sensation of thirst and declining urinary concentrating ability, which may be due to poor renal response to the antidiuretic hormone (ADH) and may be related to the decreased number of nephrons in the kidney. Therefore assessing for fluid imbalance in infants and the elderly becomes especially important.

219 You may recall that the chief sources of fluid in health are

ingestion of liquids

a _____

water in solids

b _____

metabolism (water of oxidation)

c _____

_____

220 Normally fluid losses occur through the gastrointestinal tract, the lungs, the skin, and the _____.

kidneys

FLUID VOLUME DEFICIT

221 A deficit in the fluid volume may occur for two reasons. It may be simply the result of an inadequate intake, or it may result from the fact that the loss (output) is increased over the intake. Water alone may be lost, but more likely electrolytes will be lost as well. The loss of one (water or electrolytes) may be greater than the loss of the other.

Water deficit may be due to

inadequate intake

a _____

excessive output

b _____

222 Whenever the loss of water from the body exceeds the intake, water is extracted from the extracellular fluid compartment. The result is that the remaining extracellular fluid becomes hypertonic in relation to the intracellular fluid.[3]

According to the law of osmosis, water can be expected to move (out of? into?) the cell.

out of

223 This results in cellular _____

dehydration or crenation

_____.

224 Since the extracellular fluid becomes hypertonic, the osmotic pressure is increased. The increase in osmotic pressure in the extracellular fluid stimulates the sensation of thirst. Elderly persons are likely to have an impaired sense of thirst and therefore may not drink enough fluid.

a When water is available and the person is able to ingest and absorb it, fluid volume deficit can be corrected by _____.

drinking water

b Elderly persons may not drink enough fluid because of an impaired sense of _____.

thirst

225 When the osmotic pressure of the cells becomes relatively less than that of the extracellular water, the posterior pituitary gland secretes more ADH.[8] When no ADH is secreted, the volume of urine excreted is five to ten times normal. Then the extracellular fluids become more concentrated. At the other extreme, when large quantities of ADH are secreted, excessive amounts of water are resorbed and the volume of urine may become less than one third the normal volume. Extracellular fluids then become more dilute.

In a fluid volume deficit, as a result of the decreased blood volume flowing through the kidneys and the increased secretion of ADH, normally functioning kidneys will excrete (more? less?) urine.

less

226 When there is a fluid volume deficit, the volume of extracellular water is decreased. This causes the adrenal glands to secrete aldosterone, which causes a retention of sodium that further increases the hypertonicity of the extracellular fluid.

Therefore cellular dehydration is (increased? decreased?).

increased

Laboratory findings

227 Because of a deficit of volume, the hematocrit (the proportion of erythrocytes to blood plasma) will be elevated. A normal hematocrit is 40% to 45% for women and 45% to 50% for men. A normal hematocrit for infants is 30% to 40%, and it is 31% to 43% for children.

In a person with a deficit of fluid volume, the hematocrit will be (higher? lower?) than normal for his age group.

higher

Table 3. Hematocrit in children

Age	
Newborn	53% to 65%
Infant	30% to 40%
Child	31% to 43%

From Behrman, R.E., and Vaughn, V.C.: Nelson textbook of pediatrics, ed. 12, Philadelphia, 1983, W.B. Saunders Co.

228 Since the volume of fluid is decreased, the ratio of sodium and other electrolytes in the plasma will be (increased? decreased?).

increased

229 The healthy kidneys adapt by excreting a small volume of concentrated urine. The normal specific gravity of urine is 1.010 to 1.025. In adults with adequate kidney function, an output of less than 500 to 800 ml in 24 hours is indicative of inadequate water intake.

Both infants and the elderly have a decreased ability to concentrate urine. Therefore they are more likely to develop a deficit of fluid volume.

Which of the following test results would indicate fluid volume deficit? (See page 13 for normal electrolyte values.)

_____ **a** Serum sodium 140 mEq

✓ _____ **b** Hematocrit 55%

✓ _____ **c** Specific gravity of urine 1.040

_____ **d** Serum chloride 103 mEq

Who of the following are most likely to be unable to concentrate urine?

✓ _____ **a** 3-month-old Jill

_____ **b** 10-year-old Angie

_____ **c** 40-year-old Mr. Brown

✓ _____ **d** 92-year-old Mrs. Graham

Signs and symptoms

230 Thirst is the earliest symptom of water deficit and occurs when the water loss is equal to about 2% of body weight.[8] This would be about 1400 ml in a person weighing 70 kg. As extracellular fluid is lost, the osmotic pressure of the remaining fluid is increased and water moves

84

from the cells into the extracellular compartment. Therefore the intracellular fluid volume is decreased. Apparently, the hypothalamus is sensitive to the decreased intracellular fluid volume and produces the sensation of thirst. Patients who are apathetic, confused, or very ill are likely to develop a water deficit. The sense of thirst may be impaired in infants, in persons with cerebral arteriosclerosis, in persons with cerebral injury, and in the elderly. Patients with an elevated temperature lose excessive amounts of water from the lungs. In patients with a tracheostomy, an accelerated pulmonary water loss is likely because the dead air fraction of the tidal volume is reduced. An excessive loss of water may occur in patients with burns. The nurse should anticipate the possible fluid volume deficit and see that adequate amounts of water are given in a palatable form.

The following are likely to need additional fluid intake:

apathetic and confused patients

a _____

_____

patients with elevated temperature

b _____

_____

tracheostomy patients

c _____

burn patients

d _____

infants

e _____

patients with cerebral injury

f _____

elderly patients

g _____

thirst

231 In an alert, competent person the earliest symptom of a fluid volume deficit is _____.

232 A fluid volume deficit is also likely to occur when swallowing is difficult or when the patient is comatose. Persons with diabetes insipidus cannot concentrate water because of a lack of ADH. Persons with intrinsic kidney disease may have an inability to conserve water. The nurse should be alert to other signs and symptoms when thirst is not indicated by the patient. When the water deficit is approximately 6% of body weight, the skin and mucous membranes may provide signs to indicate the fluid volume status.[8] In a person weighing 70 kg, this would be a deficit of about 4200 ml. Dry, cracked mucous membranes are indicative of an inadequate fluid intake. However, a dry and fissured tongue may also occur in a person who is a mouth breather or is receiving oxygen by mask. The skin may be flushed, and perspiration decreased. There is little saliva, and the urine output is decreased to less than 500 ml in 24 hours. Thirst is a symptom of fluid volume deficit in alert persons. The nurse should also be aware of signs of fluid volume deficit.

Which of the following signs may indicate fluid deficit?

_____ **a** Moist, clean mucous membranes
✓ _____ **b** Urine output of 400 ml in 24 hours
_____ **c** Cool, moist skin
✓ _____ **d** Dry, fissured tongue

233 If, in addition to the signs just mentioned, the patient has marked physical weakness and confusion or delirium, the water deficit is likely to be 7% to 14% of body weight. In a patient weighing 70 kg, this would be approximately 5000 to 10,000 ml.[8] The blood pressure will also decrease.

Signs of severe water deficit include

weakness   **a** _____

delirium or confusion   **b** _____

decreased blood pressure   **c** _____

234 In infants a fluid volume deficit is a very common problem that is often caused by gastroenteritis. Since an infant has a relatively greater body surface area, large quantities of fluid can be lost through the skin. Remember (frame 87) that infants ingest and excrete a greater amount of fluid per kilogram of body weight than do older children or adults.

greater   **a** An infant has a relatively (smaller? greater?) body surface area than an adult.

b Infants can lose a significant quantity of fluid through
skin   the _____.

235 Dehydration (fluid volume deficit) is one of the most common body fluid disturbances in infants and children.

Whenever the output of fluid exceeds the intake, dehydration occurs.

The most common body fluid disturbance in infants
is _____.

dehydration

236 There are three types of dehydration: isotonic, hypotonic, and hypertonic. In isotonic dehydration there is a loss of fluid and electrolytes in approximately balanced proportion. Most of the loss is sustained from the extracellular compartment.

In iostonic dehydration there is a loss of both electrolytes and _____.

fluid

237 Isotonic dehydration is the most common type of dehydration. Another type is hypotonic dehydration. Hypotonic dehydration means that the electrolyte deficit is greater than the fluid deficit. Since the extracellular fluid is hypotonic, there is movement of extracellular fluid into the intracellular space. Therefore the extracellular fluid volume becomes even less. The physical signs and symptoms tend to be more severe with hypotonic dehydration.

In hypotonic dehydration the deficit of electrolytes is (less? greater?) than the deficit of fluid.

greater

238 The third type of dehydration is hypertonic. As you can guess, hypertonic dehydration means that the deficit of fluid is greater than the deficit of electrolytes. Since fluid will then shift out of the intracellular space and into the extracellular space, the physical signs and symptoms of fluid volume deficit are not as apparent, but neurological disturbances become evident.

a In hypertonic dehydration fluid shifts (into? out of?) the extracellular compartment.

into

b In hypertonic dehydration the physical signs and symptoms of fluid volume deficit are (more? less?) apparent than in hypotonic dehydration.

less

239 Since infants and small children are unable to describe their symptoms, the nurse must be observant to detect changes (see Table 4). In isotonic and hypotonic

Table 4. Physical signs of dehydration

	Isotonic (loss of water and salt)	Hypotonic (loss of salt in excess of water)	Hypertonic (loss of water in excess of salt)
Skin			
Color	Gray	Gray	Gray
Temperature	Cold	Cold	Cold or hot
Turgor	Poor	Very poor	Fair
Feel	Dry	Clammy	Thickened
Mucous membranes	Dry	Slightly moist	Parched
Tearing and saliva-tion	Absent	Absent	Absent
Eyeball	Sunken and soft	Sunken and soft	Sunken
Fontanel	Sunken	Sunken	Sunken
Body temperature	Subnormal or elevated	Abnormal	Subnormal or elevated
Pulse	Rapid	Very rapid	Moderately rapid
Respirations	Rapid	Rapid	Rapid
Behavior	Irritable to lethargic	Lethargic to comatose; convulsions	Marked lethargy with extreme hyperirritability on stimulation

From Whaley, L.F., and Wong, D.L.: Nursing care of infants and children, ed. 3, St. Louis, 1987, The C.V. Mosby Co.

dehydration, skin turgor is lost. However, in hypertonic dehydration the skin will feel firm.

In isotonic dehydration skin turgor is (lost? firm?).

lost

240 The mucous membranes become dry with isotonic dehydration. The eyeballs appear sunken and soft. The fontanel becomes sunken or depressed. The infant's pulse and respirations are rapid.

Which of the following may indicate an isotonic dehydration?

_____ **a** Moist, mucous membranes

✓   _____ **b** Soft, sunken eyeballs

✓   _____ **c** Depressed fontanel

_____ **d** Slow pulse and respirations

241 Another significant change is a decrease in weight from the pre-illness weight. The urine output will also

Palpating anterior fontanel. (From Whaley, L.F., and Wong, D.L.: Nursing care of infants and children, ed. 3, St. Louis, 1987, The C.V. Mosby Co.)

decrease, along with an increase in specific gravity. Any other sign or symptom must also be recorded and reported.

a With a fluid volume deficit, the infant's weight will

decrease   _____.

increase   **b** The specific gravity of the urine will _____.

From Perry, A.G., and Potter, P.A.: Clinical nursing skills and techniques, St. Louis, 1986, The C.V. Mosby Co.

242 Dehydration is the most common cause of fluid and electrolyte disturbance in the elderly. This is partially due to the decrease in total body water and to the reduced thirst, along with the reduction in urinary concentrating ability that occurs with increasing age.

decreased

a One cause for dehydration in the elderly is (increased? decreased?) thirst.

less

b With increasing age, the kidneys become (less? more?) able to concentrate urine.

243 In the elderly, tissue turgor decreases with the loss of subcutaneous fat, which results in wrinkling of the skin. This should not be interpreted as a sign of dehydration.

is not

Wrinkled skin in the elderly (is? is not?) always a sign of dehydration.

Overhydration

244 Another cause of fluid volume deficit is giving large amounts of fluid to the patient too rapidly. We could suppose that giving water when there is a fluid volume deficit would correct the imbalance. However, this is true only within limits. If a very large volume of fluid is given intravenously or if the person drinks an excessively large volume of water, the urine output may be greatly increased.

volume

Although not a common cause, a deficit of fluid _____ can be produced by giving *excessive* amounts of water.

SUMMARY

Whenever the loss of water from the body exceeds the intake, water is extracted from the extracellular fluid compartment. Since the extracellular fluid becomes hypertonic, the osmotic pressure is increased and thirst results. The nurse must be alert to conditons in which water deficit could exist and observe and report any signs and/or symptoms. Marked physical weakness and confusion are signs of severe water deficit.

1 When the volume of fluid is decreased, the concentration of sodium and other electrolytes in the plasma will

increased   be _____.

2 When there is a deficit in the fluid volume, the hematocrit will be _____.

elevated

3 The following are likely to need additional fluid:

apathetic, confused, and   **a** _____
very ill patients   _____

patients with elevated tem-   **b** _____
perature   _____

tracheostomy patients   **c** _____

burn patients   **d** _____

infants   **e** _____

patients with cerebral injury   **f** _____

4 Signs of fluid deficit include the following:

dry, cracked mucous   **a** _____
membranes   _____

flushed skin   **b** _____

decreased urine output   **c** _____

5 Signs of fluid deficit in an infant include the following:

eyeballs sunken and soft   **a** _____

fontanel sunken or depressed   **b** _____

rapid pulse and respirations   **c** _____

weight loss   **d** _____

Fluid requirements

245 Average fluid requirements for adults

Intake

Ingested liquids	1500 ml
Water in foods	700 ml
Water formed in metabolism	200 ml
TOTAL	2400 ml

Output

Kidneys	
Urine	1400 ml

Lungs	
Water in expired air	350 ml
Skin	
Diffusion	350 ml
Perspiration	100 ml
Intestine	
Feces	200 ml
TOTAL	2400 ml

In a person with normally functioning kidneys, the volume of urine output is a good clue to the adequacy of the fluid intake.

The average volume of urine per 24 hours for an adult is approximately _____ ml.

1400

246 An average adult requires approximately 1500 to 2000 ml of water per day. If a person has a marked elevation of temperature, an additional 500 to 1500 ml of water is necessary daily.[8]

Therefore a person with an elevated temperature will need from _____ ml of water over a 24-hour period.

2000 to 3500

247 If a person is perspiring moderately, an additional 500 ml of water is needed. If the perspiration is profuse, another 1000 ml of water is necessary.

A person who has a temperature of 104° F and is perspiring profusely may need _____ ml of fluid over a 24-hour period.

3000 to 4500

248 Other causes for increased loss of fluid include vomiting, diarrhea, gastrointestinal drainage, burn exudate, internal pooling, wound exudate, etc.

A fluid volume deficit can be the result of an inadequate intake or an _____.

excessive or increased loss

249 Average fluid requirements for children are given in Table 5, and urine output is indicated in the box.

In a child the average output is approximately half that of an adult.

Table 5. Fluid intake

Weight	Kilogram body weight formula	Example weight	Example total fluid per 24 hr
Newborn	60–100 ml/kg	3 kg	180–300 ml
0–10 kg	100 ml/kg	8 kg	800 ml
11–20 kg	1000 ml for first 10 kg, plus 50 ml/kg over 10 kg	15 kg	1250 ml
21–30 kg	1500 ml for first 20 kg, plus 25 ml/kg over 20 kg	25 kg	1625 ml

In part from Hazinski, M.F.: Nursing care of the critically ill child, St. Louis, 1984, The C.V. Mosby Co.

Urine output

Newborn	50–300 ml/24 hr
Infant	350–500 ml/24 hr
Child	500–700 ml/24 hr
Adolescent	700–1400 ml/24 hr

From Behrman, R.E., and Vaughn, V.C.: Nelson textbook of pediatrics, ed. 12, Philadelphia, 1983, W.B. Saunders Co.

700

The average volume of urine per 24 hours for a child is approximately 500 to _____ ml.

250 The average newborn infant requires 60 to 100 ml/kg of fluid over a 24-hour period, which would be approximately 240 ml/24 hr for a 3 kg (7 pound) infant.

A 3 kg newborn infant would require approximately

240

_____ ml of fluid over a 24-hour period.

251 Fluid needs in children are based on their weight.

A 3-year-old child weighing 15 kg (33 pounds) would

1250

require approximately _____ ml of fluid over a 24-hour period.

252 If an infant or child has an elevated temperature and is perspiring, a proportionate increase will need to be added to his maintenance fluid requirements.

A child with an elevated temperature and who is perspiring will need (an increased? a decreased?) amount of fluid.

an increased

253 In the elderly there is a decrease in the total amount of body fluid; therefore their need for liquid intake is slightly less than that of younger adults. However, since aging kidneys are less able to concentrate urine, their output will remain high and will require an equal amount of intake.

Even though the total body water is less in the elderly, their intake and output (do? do not?) change significantly from younger adults.

do not

Treatment

254 Pure or distilled water can be given only orally. For many persons a water deficit can be prevented by providing adequate amounts of water in a clean, palatable form. The most satisfactory way is for the patient to drink from a glass or cup while in the sitting position. For alert patients this may be all that is necessary to increase fluid intake. Some patients especially infants, children, and elderly persons, may require assistance. For patients who must remain supine, their heads should be turned to the side if possible. Some patients should be given an explanation of how much fluid intake is desirable and why.

The most satisfactory way to provide for fluid intake for children and adults is _____
_____.

drinking from a glass while sitting up

Fluids by infusion

255 Water can be given orally except when fluids by mouth are contraindicated.

We established earlier (frame 60) that distilled water cannot be infused, because it is hypotonic and cells would _____ and _____.

swell; burst

256 The physician determines which fluids will be given parenterally. However, fluids given intravenously should be isotonic or only slightly hypotonic or hypertonic.

When fluids are given intravenously, they should be (hypotonic? isotonic? hypertonic?) to the extracellular fluid.

isotonic

257 The potential danger to the patient is increased when fluids are given intravenously. Fluids given intravenously go immediately into the systemic circulation. Although the physician is responsible for the prescription of the amount, character, and route of administration of the patient's intake, the nurse is usually responsible for the administration of the fluids. Therefore the nurse must know how to give fluids in a safe and effective manner. As with any medication, the nurse must be sure that the patient gets the correct solution, the proper amount, and at the rate prescribed. The nurse must also see that sterility of the solution and the equipment is maintained.

administration

The nurse is responsible for (prescription? administration?) of fluids.

258 In giving any medication, the nurse checks that the right drug in the proper dose, time, and method of administration is given to the right patient.

To give intravenous fluids safely and effectively, the nurse should identify the patient and see that he gets the

solution; amount
rate

right _____ , in the proper _____ at the _____ prescribed.

259 All patients should be observed regularly when fluids are given parenterally. The nurse should not rely on the patient to check the rate of infusion. The patient has neither the training nor the experience to know what to look for. The patient's energy should be conserved for recovery. Observation is especially important in patients whose homeostatic mechanisms are inadequate or defective. Patients with limited renal and/or cardiac reserve are in danger of pulmonary edema or congestive heart failure. Very young as well as older patients are less able to tolerate large volumes of fluid given rapidly. The nurse is responsible for the safe administration of fluids.

Pulmonary edema or congestive heart failure is more

95

likely to occur in patients with limited _____ and/or
_____ reserve.

260 The nurse should be alert to symptoms that indicate
congestive heart failure. If the patient becomes short of
breath, the flow rate should be decreased and the physician notified. An increase in the respiratory rate, the
occurrence of coughing, or the development of cyanosis
suggests an overloading of the patient's circulation,
with movement of fluid into the alveoli of the lungs.

Pulmonary edema and congestive heart failure are
likely to be accompanied by the following symptoms:

shortness of breath   **a** _____

increased respiratory rate   **b** _____

coughing   **c** _____

cyanosis   **d** _____

261 The rate of administration of intravenous fluids depends on the need for fluids and the nature of the fluid.
The physician will prescribe exactly how fast the fluid
should be given intravenously. The rate of flow will affect
the safety and the state of comfort of the patient. Fluids
given over a 12- to 24-hour period contribute more to the
patient's comfort and to fluid and electrolyte balance than
do fluids administered over a shorter period. The rate of
flow affects the value of the fluids to the patient.

12 to 24   Fluids given over a period of (4 to 12? 12 to 24?) hours
will be safest and most effective.

262 The rate of administration varies with the condition
of the patient and the nature of the fluid. However, the
patient must be observed frequently. Shortness of breath
may indicate that the rate is too rapid. The nurse must
be alert to the patent's urinary output in relation to the
fluid intake and observe and report signs of too rapid a
rate of administration.

A patient who is receiving intravenous fluids and who
becomes short of breath should have the rate of fluid flow
decreased   (increased? left the same? decreased?).

263 When fluids are being given intravenously to infants

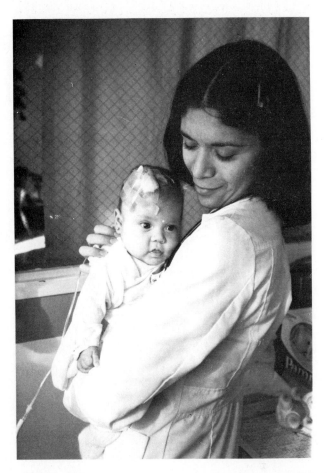

Intravenous infusion does not prevent infant from being picked up and cuddled. (From Whaley, L.F., and Wong, D.L.: Nursing care of infants and children, ed. 3, St. Louis, 1987, The C.V. Mosby Co.)

and children, accurate intake is essential. The rate of administration of the fluids must be kept constant. Therefore some type of volume control device is used with infants and children (see the illustration on page 98). Even a very small error could cause serious problems. Rates in children generally vary from 5 to 80 ml/hr depending on the size of the child, whereas the rate for an adolescent or adult could be 80 to 150 ml/hr.

The rate for intravenous fluids in a child varies from _____ to 80 ml/hr.

5

From Perry, A.G., and Potter, P.A.: *Clinical nursing skills and techniques*, St. Louis, 1986, The C.V. Mosby Co.

Calculating the rate of flow

264 The rate of administration of fluids intravenously can be calculated when we know the drop size for the administration set we are using. The size of the drops varies in the different parenteral administration sets. We should know how many drops are needed to give 1 ml (1 cc) with the administration set being used. The variation in size of drops with different commercial administration sets is as follows:

Approximate no. of drops to deliver 1 ml

Company	Regular set	Pediatric set
Abbott	15	60
Baxter	10	50
Cutter	20	60

When we divide the number of drops per minute by the number of drops per milliliter that our administration set gives, we find the number of milliliters per minute. To find how many milliliters are being given per hour, we then multiply by 60 (60 minutes = 1 hour). If we were using an Abbott set, which requires 15 drops for each milliliter, we would use the drops per minute, divide by

15, and then multiply by 60. We may arrive at the same figure if we use a shortcut that Goldberger calls the drop factor[8]: we divide 60 (the minutes in 1 hour) by 15 (the number of drops per milliliter) to get 4. In this example, 4 is our drop factor; to find the milliliters per hour, we multiply the drops per minute by the drop factor.

a If the administration set requires 15 drops for 1 ml of fluid and the fluid is flowing at 25 drops/min, the patient will be receiving _____ /hr.

25 × 4 = 100 ml

b If we use a drop factor of 4 and the rate is 35 drops/ min, the patient will receive _____ /hr.

35 × 4 = 140 ml

c If we use a Baxter administration set, requiring 10 drops for 1 ml, our drop factor will be _____.

60 ÷ 10 = 6

265 Now suppose we are to give 1000 ml of fluid in 8 hours. We need to know first how many milliliters per hour are desired.

a 1000 ml ÷ 8 = _____ ml/hr.

125

   The drops per minute necessary are found by dividing the milliliters per hour by the drop factor.

b If the administration set requires 15 drops/ml, the drop factor will be _____.

60 ÷ 15 = 4

c The number of drops per minute necessary to give 1000 ml of fluid in 8 hours is _____.

125 ml ÷ 4 = 31

266 We have an order to give 4000 ml of fluid in 24 hours.

   If the administration set requires 15 drops/ml, how shall we calculate the drops per minute required to give 4000 ml in 24 hours? (Round off fractions to nearest whole number.)

4000 ÷ 24 = 167 ml/hr
60 ÷ 15 = 4 (drop factor)
167 ÷ 4 = 42 drops/min

a _____

b _____

c _____

267 To check our answer, we multiply the drops per minute by the drop factor to get the milliliters per hour.

a 42 × 4 = _____.

168

   We then multiply the milliliters per hour times the number of hours.

b 168 × 24 = _____.

4032

Mechanical factors affecting flow rate

268 A change in the position of the needle may alter the rate of flow. If the bevel of the needle is against the wall of the vein, the rate will be slower than normal. A change in the height of the bottle of fluid above the needle site in the patient will alter the rate. The greater the height of the bottle above the needle site in the patient, the faster will be the rate of flow.

If we raise the bottle of fluid higher, the rate of flow will (increase? not change? decrease?).

increase

269 If we keep the bottle of fluid the same height above the floor and raise the level of the patient's bed, the flow rate will _____.

decrease

270 The patency of the needle will alter the flow rate. A change in position of the limb may affect the rate.

Mechanical factors that influence the flow rate of intravenous fluids include the following:.

change in needle position

a _____

patency of needle

b _____

change in position of limb

c _____

change in height of bottle above patient

d _____

_____

Adjusting rate of flow

271 Since the intravenous infusion is most effective when spaced over a long period of time, the infusion rate must remain nearly constant (except in emergency situations). However, after the rate is adjusted, continuous supervision is required to see that it does not change because of mechanical factors. In adults the rate should be checked at least every hour. In infants and children the rate should be counted and recorded every 15 minutes.

a In children the rate of intravenous infusion should be counted every _____ minutes.

15

b In adults, the rate of intravenous infusion should be counted every _____.

hour

Rate of infusion should be checked by watch. (From Perry, A.G., and Potter, P.A.: Clinical nursing skills and techniques, St. Louis, 1986, The C.V. Mosby Co.)

272 If a liter of fluid is to be given over a period of 8 to 12 hours, the bottle should be labeled as to how many milliliters per hour are to be administered ("1000 ml 5% dextrose in saline to run for 8 hours"). In this way the nurse can tell quite accurately whether the rate is still adjusted correctly. A piece of adhesive or masking tape can be used to indicate the milliliters to be given per hour and where the level of fluid should be each hour. Although this method works best on a glass or rigid container, an approximate level can be indicated on any container.

a If 1000 ml is started at 7 AM and is to be given over a period of 8 hours, _____ milliliters should be given by 11 AM.

500

b By 1 PM, _____ should be given.

750 ml

273 Hypertonic and hypotonic solutions should be given at a slower rate than isotonic solutions. One of the best guides to a safe rate of flow is the reaction of the patient. Therefore the nurse must observe signs and symptoms carefully.

Symptoms of pulmonary edema include the following:

a _____

b _____

c _____

d _____

shortness of breath
coughing
cyanosis
increased respiratory rate

274 If these symptoms occur, the nurse should

a _____

b _____

(Refer to frame 260 if necessary.)

slow the rate of infusion
notify the physician

275 If the patient becomes short of breath, the rate of infusion should be (slowed? increased?).

slowed

276 The maximum rate for administration of glucose to normal adults without producing glycosuria is approximately 0.5 g per kilogram of body weight per hour (0.5 g/kg/hr).[3] At this rate it would take approximately 1½ hours to administer 1000 ml of 5% dextrose in water or saline solution to a patient weighing 70 kg (154 pounds), or twice as long for 1000 ml of 10% dextrose. The exact rate at which fluids are to be infused should be determined by the physician. A safe method of determining the rate of fluid administration is to divide the volume of fluid to be given by 24 hours.

The safest method of fluid administration is to give the fluids over a _____ period.

24-hour

277 If the rate of infusion exceeds the suggested maximum rate, the body is unable to metabolize the glucose. Therefore it is excreted in the urine. This further increases the output of fluid, since more fluid is required in which to dilute the glucose for excretion.

The maximum rate at which the body can metabolize glucose is _____ g per kilogram of body weight per hour.

0.5

SUMMARY

The volume of urine output serves as a good indication of the adequacy of fluid intake in anyone with normally functioning kidneys. When there is a fluid volume deficit, fluids can be given orally or parenterally. The nurse is responsible for the administration of fluids and must be alert to the dangers when fluids are given parenterally. Dyspnea, increased respiratory rate, coughing, and cyanosis are symptoms that indicate an overload of the patient's circulatory system. Since the patient will benefit more from an intravenous infusion if it is spaced over a longer period of time, the nurse must know how to calculate and adjust the rate of flow.

REVIEW

1 At the morning report you are told that Mr. Green, a 53-year-old man who has had a cerebral vascular accident, had a urine output of 400 ml for the past 24 hours.

24-hour intake

Next you should find out his _____.

2 Mrs. Cole, a 90-year-old woman who was admitted yesterday, is receiving fluids intravenously. You note that her respiratory rate is increasing and she is beginning to cough frequently.

slow the rate of infusion

Your first action should be to _____ _____.

3 Mr. Berry, who has had a cerebral vascular accident and is unable to swallow, is to receive 3000 ml of fluid intravenously. He will get the most benefit from the fluids if they are (spaced over a 24-hour period? run very rapidly?).

spaced over a 24-hour period

4 Rosa, 7 months, was admitted to the hospital because of dehydration. The physician has ordered the intravenous infusion to run at 50 ml/hr. You should check the rate of flow every _____.

15 minutes

FLUID VOLUME EXCESS

278 Just as it is possible to develop a fluid volume deficit, so it is possible to have an excess of extracellular fluid volume. Fluid volume excess is not likely to occur unless the renal mechanisms fail. The cause of fluid excess may be diseased kidneys, excessive secretion of ADH, or decreased blood flow through the kidneys. Decreased blood flow through the kidneys is likely to occur in elderly persons. The cause of fluid excess is the same in children as in adults. As in fluid volume deficit, the electrolytes are out of balance along with fluid volume excess. When there is an increase in the extracellular fluid volume, the osmotic pressure is reduced because there is a decrease in the number of particles per unit of water.[3] As a consequence, fluid moves from the extracellular compartment into the cell.

swell

Therefore the cells (swell? shrink?).

279 Normally, when a person takes an excess of water and water moves into the cells, this causes the osmoreceptors to respond and the posterior pituitary decreases the secretion of ADH. As a result, the excess fluid is excreted by the kidneys. However, if a patient has an excessive secretion of ADH, then the water will be retained. Therefore more fluid will move into the cells.

less

Normally, excess fluid in the cells causes the posterior pituitary to secrete (more? less?) ADH.

280 When the secretion of ADH is decreased, the urinary output is (increased? decreased?).

increased

281 There are several reasons why a patient may have excessive secretion of ADH. Excessive secretion of ADH can occur as a result of fear, pain, or acute infections. It can also occur as a result of most anesthetics or analgesics such as morphine or meperidine hydrochloride (Demerol). Any acute stress (such as trauma or a major operation) may stimulate excessive secretion of ADH. Postoperatively the excessive secretion of ADH may last 12 to 36 hours or longer.[3] Oxytocin has antidiuretic properties and may cause volume excess if injected along with an infusion of dextrose and water.[8] Accurate measurement of intake, output, and the patient's weight is important after any acute stress.

increase

a The effect of stress on the secretion of ADH is to (increase? decrease?) secretion.

decreased

b This results in (increased? decreased?) excretion of fluid.

282 An excessive secretion of ADH is likely to occur in which of the following situations?

✓ _____ **a** Twenty-four hours after cholecystectomy

✓ _____ **b** A patient who had a coronary occlusion yesterday and continues to have severe pain

✓ _____ **c** A patient who is receiving meperidine, 100 mg every 3 hours, for pain from a ureteral calculus

_____ **d** A patient who had a fractured femur pinned 10 days ago

✓ _____ **e** A postpartum patient who was hemorrhaging and was given oxytocin in an intravenous solution of 5% dextrose in water

283 Some persons with cerebral lesions or lung cancer may have excessive secretion of ADH.

As the secretion of ADH increases, the excretion of

decreases

urine _____.

284 Whenever there is a low renal blood flow and the kidneys are unable to excrete urine, fluid volume excess is likely to occur. In persons with adrenal cortical insufficiency or acute renal insufficiency, excessive retention of water occurs because the kidneys do not excrete water. In severe congestive heart failure or cirrhosis of the liver the renal blood flow is low. Therefore the kidneys are unable to excrete normal amounts of fluid.

An excess of fluid volume is likely to occur in a person with severe congestive heart failure because of the decreased renal blood flow, which results in (increased? unchanged? decreased?) urinary output.

285 Water excess can occur if large volumes of water are given rectally because the water comes in contact with the absorbing surface of the colon. Patients who have lost sodium are likely to develop water excess because the osmotic pressure of the extracellular fluid is lower than that of the cells.

Giving large amounts of water rectally may result in fluid volume (excess? deficit?).

Signs and symptoms

286 Fluid volume excess can be prevented if the nurse carefully observes and reports the patient's total fluid intake and output. Changes in the patient's weight can provide data that, when added to other facts, will indicate the fluid volume status. For each pound of weight gained, about 1 pint of fluid (500 ml) is retained. An acute weight gain, in excess of 5% of body weight, may indicate fluid excess.[5]

a In a person weighing 150 pounds, this would be a weight gain of _____ pounds.

b An acute gain in weight may be indicative of fluid volume (excess? deficit?).

c When there is a fluid volume deficit, the extracellular fluid becomes (hypotonic? isotonic? hypertonic?).

d When there is a fluid volume excess, the extracellular fluid becomes _____.

e When the extracellular fluid is hypotonic, fluid will move (into? out of?) the cell.

287 As fluid moves into the cells, the cells swell. The symptoms that patients have in fluid volume excess are the result of disturbed cerebral function. In severe fluid volume excess the patient develops unusual behavior, loss of attention, confusion, and aphasia. This may be followed by convulsions, coma, and death.[3]

In fluid volume excess, symptoms due to disturbed cerebral function include

a _____

loss of attention   **b** _____

confusion   **c** _____

aphasia   **d** _____

288 In fluid volume excess the skin is warm and moist and may be flushed. The cardiovascular system remains normal as long as the excess fluid volume remains in the interstitial spaces or does not become too great. Edema may occur in dependent parts of the body or in the lungs, especially if the person has congestive heart failure.

Which of the following may indicate fluid volume excess?

✓   _____ **a** Warm moist skin

_____ **b** Cool dry skin

✓   _____ **c** Mental confusion

_____ **d** Loss of weight

✓   _____ **e** Convulsions

289 In a person with congestive heart failure who has a fluid volume excess, the likely symptoms include edema of dependent body parts and lungs. Symptoms of edema or fluid in the lungs are the same as those discussed in fluid volume deficit when fluid is given too rapidly and pulmonary edema results. Also, the blood pressure may rise.

Symptoms of pulmonary edema include the following:

shortness of breath   **a** _____

coughing   **b** _____

cyanosis   **c** _____

increased respiratory rate   **d** _____

decreased   **290** The hemoglobin and hematocrit levels are (increased? decreased?) because of the fluid volume excess.

291 The mean corpuscular volume (MCV) of the erythrocytes is increased because the osmotic pressure in the extracellular fluid is lower than that of the cells.

drawn into   Therefore water is (drawn into? pushed out of?) the cells.

292 If a postoperative patient develops unusual behavior, has a convulsive seizure, experiences hemiplegia, or becomes comatose, fluid volume excess should be suspected. The water-excess syndrome that follows surgery or trauma is usually self-limited. However, if the person has a convulsion or hemiplegia or becomes comatose, death may follow even though active treatment is given.

It is especially important for the nurse to keep an accurate record of fluid intake and output as well as weight of patients in the first few days after surgery or trauma, for these persons are susceptible to fluid volume

excess   _____.

293 Convulsions or hemiplegia caused by fluid volume

serious   excess are indicative of (self-limited? serious?) fluid volume excess.

Treatment

294 Fluid volume excess may be treated by limiting the fluid intake. How much the fluid intake is restricted depends on the condition of the patient. If the patient has renal failure, the fluid intake may be limited to 300 to 500 ml in 24 hours.[3] If the patient has had a convulsion or is experiencing hemiplegia, fluids must be withheld and a hypertonic saline solution should be given.[8] In infants and children a proportionate amount of fluids should be withheld.

In an adult, in acute renal failure the fluid intake may

300 to 500   be limited to _____ ml in 24 hours.

295 If the fluid volume excess is serious, the fluid intake

stopped   may be (restricted? stopped?).

296 Any acute stress may stimulate an excessive secre-

excess   tion of ADH, which can lead to fluid volume (excess? deficit?).

297 This can be corrected before the excess becomes serious if the nurse daily collects the following data in susceptible persons:

intake   **a** _____

output   **b** _____

weight   **c** _____

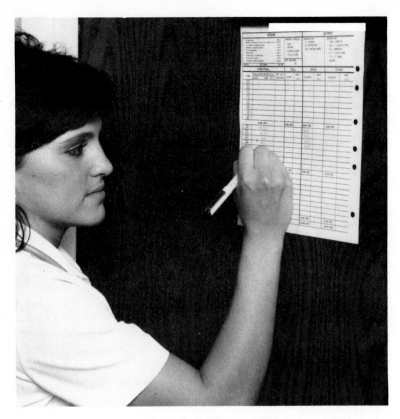

From Perry, A.G., and Potter, P.A.: Clinical nursing skills and techniques, St. Louis, 1986, The C.V. Mosby Co.

SUMMARY

Normally, when excess fluid moves into cells, the secretion of ADH is decreased; therefore the urine output is increased. However, any acute stress may stimulate an excessive secretion of ADH, which results in decreased excretion of fluid. In fluid volume excess, symptoms caused by disturbed cerebral function include confusion, loss of attention, unusual behavior, and aphasia. These may be followed by convulsions, coma, and death. The nurse must carefully observe patients likely to develop fluid volume excess and keep records of

109

intake, output, and weight. In this way the excess fluid volume may be corrected before it becomes serious.

REVIEW

1 Mr. Short weighed 171 pounds yesterday. Today his weight is 180 pounds. After determining that this is his actual weight today, the nurse should be aware that the gain may represent _____.

fluid volume excess

2 The nurse should look for symptoms due to fluid volume excess. Symptoms of disturbed cerebral function include the following:

unusual behavior   **a** _____

loss of attention   **b** _____

confusion   **c** _____

aphasia   **d** _____

warm and moist

3 In fluid volume excess the skin will be _____
_____.

restrict

4 The first step in treating fluid volume excess is to _____ fluid intake.

FLUID VOLUME SHIFTS

298 Fluids may shift from the intravascular compartments into the interstitial space. In some clinical disorders, depletion of the extracellular fluid develops because large quantities of fluid are held in an interstitial area, which makes them inaccessible to the body. This is called "third spacing," and the fluid is usually essentially invisible.

The term "third spacing" refers to fluids that are (available? not available?) for use by the body.

not available

299 This shift of fluid into "third space" may be localized to a single area or organ, or it can spread throughout the body. For example, a person with ascites will have large quantities of fluid in the abdomen. A person who has had abdominal surgery may have significant quantities of fluid that are not available for use by the body. The reasons why fluids may shift into "third space" includes lowered plasma proteins, increased capillary permeability, or lymphatic blockage. These changes in the movement of fluids may be secondary to trauma, inflammation, or disease. It is a major factor in the fluid balance of persons who have had abdominal surgery.

The factors that allow fluids to move from the intravascular compartment into "third space" include

decreased   **a** (decreased? increased?) plasma proteins

increased   **b** (decreased? increased?) capillary permeability

lymphatic   **c** _____ blockage

300 The first phase of "third spacing" is loss. Depending on the cause, it is likely to last for 48 to 72 hours. During this time the symptoms will be those of a fluid volume deficit.

In the first phase of "third spacing" you should expect symptoms of fluid volume (excess? deficit?).

deficit

301 During this phase, fluids shift from the vascular to the interstitial spaces. The shift in fluids occurs because of increased capillary permeability in areas of inflammation and trauma. The increased capillary permeability allows plasma proteins to leak into the interstitial space. In some situations lymphatic blockage may allow fluid to remain in the interstitial spaces. When fluids shift into "third space" even though intravenous fluids are being given, the fluid does not stay in the intravascular compartment and the patient becomes hypovolemic. The person has a decreased blood volume.

When fluids shift into "third space," the blood volume or intravascular fluid volume decreases. This is called

hypovolemia   _____.

302 The clinical signs you should watch for with hypovolemia include a decreased blood pressure and an increased heart rate.

decrease   **a** In hypovolemia the blood pressure will (increase? decrease?).

increase   **b** The heart rate will (increase? decrease?).

303 You will expect to find an increase in heart rate and a decrease in blood pressure when hypovolemia occurs.

Also, a person with hypovolemia will have a low central venous pressure and a decreased urine output.

a In hypovolemia the central venous pressure will be (high? normal? low?).

low

decrease

b The urine output will (increase? decrease?).

304 The second phase of "third spacing" is resorption. After the inflammation subsides, the fluid in the tissue spaces begins to be resorbed. Therefore intravascular volume will increase. Usually this shift occurs gradually and fluid overload does not occur unless extra fluid is given at this time.

The second phase of "third spacing" is resorption; fluid moves into the _____ compartment.

intravascular

305 During the resorption phase, nursing observations and actions should be the same as those in fluid volume excess The information the nurse should collect daily in susceptible persons is

intake

a _____

output

b _____

weight

c _____

SUMMARY

Following trauma, inflammation, or some diseases, fluid may shift from the intravascular compartment into the interstitial compartment and is not accessible to the body. This is called "third spacing." The first phase of "third spacing" is loss, and it may last for 48 to 72 hours. During this time the symptoms are those of fluid volume deficit. The second phase of "third spacing" is resorption. Usually this shift of fluids back into the intravascular space is gradual. Nursing care is aimed at observations and actions to prevent severe fluid volume deficit during the first phase and to prevent fluid volume excess during the resorption phase. The nurse must be sure to keep accurate records of intake, output, and weight. An accurate intake and output is especially important for infants and for elderly persons.

REVIEW

1 When "third spacing" occurs during the first phase, the shift of fluid is (out of? into?) the intravascular compartment.

out of

2 During the first 48 to 72 hours following trauma or inflammation, the symptoms are those of fluid volume _____.

deficit

3 The second phase of "third spacing" usually involves the movement of fluids into the _____ space.

intravascular

4 While caring for infants or elderly persons with "third spacing," the nurse should keep careful records of _____, _____, and _____.

intake; output; weight

CASE STUDIES

Lisa Davis

1 Lisa Davis, a 4-month-old infant, has been admitted to the hospital with a history of vomiting and diarrhea for 5 days. She is dehydrated and has a rectal temperature of 104° F. Her skin is dry, and her respirations are rapid and shallow, with a rate of 68/min. Her apical heart rate is 164 beats/min. Her fontanel is depressed. An intravenous infusion has been started in a scalp vein. Lisa's vomiting and frequent loose stools continue.

decreased

a You would expect her weight to be (increased? decreased?) from her pre-illness weight.

increased

b You would expect her serum sodium level to be (increased? decreased?) from the normal.

2 Lisa has a convulsion, and her respirations drop to 4/min. She has an endotracheal tube inserted and is put on a ventilator.

severe

Her fluid volume deficit is (mild? severe?).

James Wentzel

1 Mr. James Wentzel, age 82, has been admitted to the hospital for possible surgery to correct a urinary tract obstruction. He has been unable to void for the past 12

113

hours and has had urgency and frequency for several weeks.

a If Mr. Wentzel has signs of water intoxication, you would expect his skin to be _____ and

cool; moist

_____.

increased

b You would expect his weight to have (increased? decreased?).

c If Mr. Wentzel has water intoxication and his extracellular fluid is hypotonic, you would expect him to

confused

be (alert? confused?).

John Winn

1 John Winn is a 22-year-old man who was hospitalized after a gunshot wound in his abdomen. Two days ago he had surgery to repair a perforated colon and duodenum. He has a nasogastric tube in place, and it is functioning well. This morning he complains of more abdominal discomfort. You notice that his abdomen is distended. When you take his vital signs, his heart rate has gone from 86 up to 116 beats/min and his blood pressure has dropped from 130/84 to 100/68.

You should think about the possibility that Mr. Winn

into the interstitial space

may have a shift of fluid _____ ,

"third spacing"

also called _____.

decreased

2 You would expect that his urine output has _____.

114

PART 4 Electrolyte imbalance

INTRODUCTION

Each electrolyte has special functions in the body. Although some electrolytes play larger roles than do others, all are necessary for the maintenance of life. There are four basic physiological processes for which electrolytes are essential: (1) promotion of neuromuscular irritability, (2) maintenance of body fluid osmolarity, (3) regulation of acid-base balance, and (4) distribution of body fluids between the fluid compartments.

We shall consider the special functions of sodium, potassium, magnesium, and calcium.

306 The physiological processes for which electrolytes are essential include the following:

neuromuscular irritability   **a** _____

body fluid osmolarity   **b** _____

acid-base balance   **c** _____

distribution of body fluids   **d** _____

SODIUM IMBALANCE

307 Sodium is the major cation in the extracellular fluid. In fact, it represents about 90% of all the extracellular cations. Sodium ions are especially important in regulating the voltage of action potentials. Sodium is necessary for the transmission of impulses in nerve and muscle fibers. For example, if there is a deficit in the sodium

115

concentration, there will be muscle weakness. Since sodium is the most osmotically active solute in the intravascular and interstitial fluid, it is one of the main factors that determine extracellular fluid volume. Sodium is primarily found outside the cell and is osmotically active. Therefore it plays a major role in controlling the size of the cell.

a Sodium is essential for the normal transmission of impulses in _____ and _____.

muscles; nerves

volume

b Sodium is also necessary to maintain the _____ of extracellular fluid.

308 The level of sodium in the body is controlled by multiple factors that are not completely understood. These factors include the adrenal glands, the pituitary gland, the skin, the gastrointestinal tract, arterial pressure, and compositional changes in the extracellular fluid. The combined effect is that the kidneys are influenced to resorb more or less sodium from the blood and to excrete it in the urine.[18] For example, if the level of sodium in the body goes down, the kidneys will excrete urine that is practically free of sodium. Active resorption of sodium by the kidneys takes place in the tubules. Normally almost all the sodium is resorbed and none of it is excreted. However, if the level of sodium is high, large portions of sodium can be excreted in the urine.

most

The normal kidneys usually resorb (most? little?) of the sodium that is filtered through them.

309 If the level of sodium becomes high, normal kidneys (can? cannot?) excrete the excess sodium.

can

310 Most of the sodium that is resorbed is associated with chloride.

Resorbed sodium is usually in the form of sodium

chloride

_____.

311 The kidneys are extremely important in regulating sodium balance, primarily through the action of aldosterone.

The hormone from the adrenal glands that is most

aldosterone

influential in regulating sodium balance is _____.

312 Normally almost all the sodium that is filtered by the kidneys is resorbed. Most of the sodium is resorbed with chloride, but some is resorbed when sodium ions are exchanged for potassium and hydrogen ions. In the absence of aldosterone, a person can become seriously depleted of sodium and chloride.

sodium

Aldosterone is an important hormone for the regulation of _____ and chloride.

313 There are several factors that affect the rate of secretion of aldosterone. Any one or a combination of these factors stimulates the secretion of aldosterone and, consequently, the level of sodium. These factors include reduced blood volume or cardiac output, decreased extracellular sodium, increased extracellular potassium, and physical stress. Renin, which is secreted by the kidneys and causes the formation of angiotensin, also may act directly on the adrenal cortex to secrete more aldosterone when the sodium concentration is low.

aldosterone

a Reduced blood volume and cardiac output stimulate the production of _____.

low

b Aldosterone is secreted in greater amounts when the level of extracellular sodium is (high? low?).

high

c The secretion of aldosterone is stimulated by a (high? low?) level of extracellular potassium.

314 In the elderly the renal blood flow decreases, the cardiac output decreases, the plasma renin activity is lower, and the stress response to sodium restriction is blunted. All of these changes that occur with aging affect the rate of secretion of aldosterone. This indicates the increased vulnerability of the elderly person to a sodium imbalance.

more

The elderly are (more? less?) likely to have a sodium imbalance than are children or younger adults.

315 The regulation of sodium in the body is very closely interwoven with the regulation of fluid volume, since the fluid volume can be adjusted by regulating the level of sodium in the body.

increase

Because of the osmolarity, as the sodium content increases, the volume of fluid will (increase? decrease?).

117

Sodium deficit

316 We shall now consider some of the causes of a sodium deficit, called *hyponatremia.* "Natrium" is the Latin word for sodium, and the symbol is Na. Though normally sodium and chloride are resorbed by the kidneys, sodium may be lost from the body through gastrointestinal secretions. Vomiting, diarrhea, or gastrointestinal drainage from suction or fistulas may cause a loss of sodium.

a loss

Loss of secretions from the gastrointestinal tract may cause (a loss? an increase?) of sodium.

317 Sodium may be lost through the skin, as in excessive sweating, burns, and cystic fibrosis.

skin

In sweating, as well as in burns and cystic fibrosis, sodium is lost through the _____.

318 Hyponatremia may also occur when sodium is isolated within the body and is not physiologically available, as when there is an obstruction of the small bowel and large amounts of fluid containing sodium are held in the intestinal lumen. It may occur in burns when edema accumulates at the burn site or in peritonitis when extracellular fluid is held in the abdomen. The sodium in these fluids is not available for necessary functions.

Fluid containing sodium may be isolated in the body when any of the following occurs:

small bowel obstruction   **a** _____

burns   **b** _____

peritonitis   **c** _____

319 Another cause of hyponatremia is renal disease, especially salt-losing nephritis.

sodium

If the kidneys are unable to resorb _____, there will be hyponatremia.

320 Although both fluid and electrolytes are lost in the previously mentioned conditions causing sodium deficit, the fluid may be more readily replaced, leaving a deficit of sodium. For example, a construction worker who is perspiring from hard work is likely to drink large quantities of water. Thus his fluid volume may be restored, but the sodium loss will not be replaced unless he also increases his intake of salt (sodium chloride).

Whenever sodium is lost from the body, the fluid volume will be (increased? decreased?).

decreased

Signs and symptoms

321 The signs and symptoms will depend on the degree of depletion of sodium and water as well as the rapidity of the loss. If the loss is severe and occurs suddenly, the clinical picture will be of shock. If the loss is more gradual, the symptoms will include weakness, apathy, and lassitude.

Weakness, apathy, and lassitude are symptoms of sodium (deficit? excess?).

deficit

322 Muscle weakness, fatigue, headache, hypotension, and vertigo may occur with a sodium deficit. Muscle cramps may occur, especially if the fluid is replaced without the sodium, since fluid replacement intensifies the sodium loss. In the elderly these symptoms are often attributed to aging, and the hypokalemia may be missed.

Headache, vertigo, hypotension, muscle weakness, and muscle _____ may occur in sodium deficit.

cramps

323 In addition to the symptoms of fatigue, apathy, and muscle weakness, a person with hyponatremia may have gastrointestinal symptoms, including anorexia, nausea, and vomiting.

A person with hyponatremia may have gastrointestinal symptoms of

anorexia   **a** _____

nausea   **b** _____

vomiting   **c** _____

324 Since the level of sodium in the body also controls the extracellular fluid volume, some of the signs and symptoms of sodium deficit will parallel those of fluid volume deficit. There will be a loss of skin turgor; that is, if the skin of the arm is picked up and released, it will

119

tend to remain stretched and folded for a half minute or more. Normally, when the skin is picked up, it returns almost immediately to its previous shape. In the elderly, skin turgor is not a useful sign of sodium deficit, since skin loses elasticity with advancing age.

turgor

In sodium deficit the skin will show loss of _____ in children and younger adults.

From Perry, A.G., and Potter, P.A.: Clinical nursing skills and techniques, St. Louis, 1986, The C.V. Mosby Co.

325 The eyeballs may be sunken and feel soft on palpation. The tongue may be wrinkled and shrunk.

In addition to a loss of skin turgor with hyponatremia, there may be changes in the eyeballs and

tongue

_____.

326 The cardiovascular signs will vary with the rate and degree of sodium loss. There may be orthostatic hypotension, which is a drop in blood pressure when the person stands and which may cause fainting.

hypotension

Hyponatremia may cause orthostatic _____.

327 There may also be tachycardia, thready peripheral pulse or loss of peripheral pulse, and collapsed neck veins.

In hyponatremia the pulse may be rapid and thready

collapse

and the neck veins may _____.

328 If the hyponatremia develops slowly or is less severe, the symptoms will be less dramatic. Be alert to the possible need for sodium in the person who is fatigued, has a loss of energy, and feels faint on arising.

Hyponatremia that is not severe may cause symptoms of

fatigue

a _____

120

loss of energy

fainting

b _____

c _____

Laboratory findings

329 The hematocrit will be elevated because of hemoconcentration, yet the serum sodium will be low. The normal level of intravascular sodium is given on page 13. In hyponatremia the serum sodium will be less than 135 mEq/L. The level of sodium does not change with increasing age. The level of sodium is useful in differentiating sodium loss from water loss. In water loss a high hematocrit level is associated with a high sodium concentration.

above

a In hyponatremia the hematocrit will be (above? below?) normal.

below

b The serum sodium will be (above? below?) normal.

330 The serum level of chloride or bicarbonate will also be low. The serum potassium may be high, since some loss of sodium will cause increased retention of potassium.

low

The serum level of chloride will likely be (high? low?).

331 In sodium deficit the urinary volume will likely be low, as will the sodium and chloride concentration in the urine.

low

The urinary volume and concentration of sodium and chloride will be (high? low?).

Treatment

332 The aim of treatment is to restore balance by replacing the deficit of sodium and water. If shock exists, parenteral sodium and water will be needed. Pressor amines such as norepinephrine (Levophed) or metaraminol (Aramine) will not be effective until some of the sodium has been replaced. A liter of isotonic saline solution (0.85%) contains 154 mEq of sodium. The amount of sodium to be replaced is calculated by the physician on the basis of the serum sodium level and the weight of the patient. The rate of flow for parenteral replacement must be carefully controlled, since too rapid replacement will increase the loss of electrolytes.

a If the hyponatremia is severe, replacement of sodium and water will be needed by the _____ route.

parenteral (intravenous)

b The rate of flow for sodium chloride solution administered intravenously should be (rapid? controlled?).

controlled

333 In less severe hyponatremia the sodium content of the patient's oral fluids may be increased.

In some conditions sodium can be replaced _____ rather than parenterally.

orally

334 Another aspect of treatment is to stop further loss of sodium. For example, if the patient is losing fluid from a pancreatic fistula, this fluid will have a high sodium content. Therefore isotonic saline solution should be used to replace the loss. Additonal sodium chloride may be necessary.

Pancreatic drainage has a high _____ content.

sodium

SUMMARY

Sodium is the main extracellular cation. Some functions of sodium are transmission of impulses in nerve and muscle fibers, control of cell size, and maintenance of extracellular fluid volume.

Normal kidneys can selectively regulate the level of sodium in the body. Reduced blood volume, decreased cardiac output, low extracellular sodium, high extracellular potassium, and physical stress stimulate the secretion of aldosterone, which causes an increased resorption of sodium by the kidneys.

All secretions from the gastrointestinal tract contain sodium, which is normally resorbed. Therefore any abnormal loss of gastrointestinal secretions can cause a sodium deficit (hyponatremia). Sodium may also be lost through the skin or through the kidneys. A sudden loss of sodium may produce shock. A gradual loss of sodium may be evidenced by symptoms of fatigue, loss of energy, and fainting. Other signs of hyponatremia include tachycardia and hypotension. The hematocrit will be above normal, and the serum sodium will be low. Treatment is aimed at restoration of balance by replacing the deficit of sodium, often in the form of sodium chloride, and the deficit of water.

REVIEW

1 The most osmotically active extracellular cation is

sodium

_____.

all

2 Normally almost (all? none?) of the sodium filtered by the kidney is resorbed.

increased

3 A reduced cardiac output will stimulate (increased? decreased?) secretion of aldosterone.

potassium; hydrogen

4 When sodium is resorbed because of the effect of aldosterone, more _____ and _____ ions are excreted.

sodium

5 In peritonitis, in which large amounts of extracellular fluid are held in the peritoneal cavity, there may be a _____ deficit, since this fluid is not available to the body.

increase the problem

6 In the treatment of a sodium deficit by the intravenous administration of sodium chloride, very rapid replacement may (be indicated? increase the problem?).

low

7 Ms. Bond, age 42, has been vomiting for 2 days. You would expect her serum sodium to be (high? normal? low?).

8 Which of the following signs or symptoms would you expect to find in Ms. Bond?

✓ ____ a Fatigue
____ b Hypertension
✓ ____ c Weakness
✓ ____ d Loss of skin turgor
____ e Edema

Sodium excess

335 The kidneys regulate the excretion of sodium in a healthy person according to intake. If the kidneys fail because of hormonal or hemodynamic effects, an excess of sodium (hypernatremia) may develop. When this occurs, there is also a retention of fluid, or edema, and therefore an increase in extracellular fluid volume. For the kidneys to perform their regulatory function, an adequate blood flow must be present, as well as a normal aldosterone system. Therefore the conditions in which hypernatremia may be a problem include renal failure (with sodium retention), inadequate circulation of blood to the kidneys (as in congestive heart failure), cirrhosis of the liver, overproduction of aldosterone by the adrenal cortex, and use of large doses of adrenal corticoids. Since these conditions may occur in the elderly, they are likely to develop sodium excess. Elderly persons may eat more convenience-type foods, which are often high in sodium.

blood flow
aldosterone

The kidneys must have adequate ＿＿＿＿＿＿ and ＿＿＿＿＿＿＿ to regulate the sodium level.

336 Even if the kidneys do resorb increased amounts of sodium, the concentration of sodium usually will not increase significantly, since the person becomes extremely thirsty and thus drinks water, which dilutes the sodium that is resorbed. Then the problem is fluid volume excess rather than sodium excess or hypernatremia.

does not increase

Usually the concentration of sodium (increases? does not increase?) significantly, even if increased amounts of sodium are resorbed.

337 We can say, then, that hypernatremia causes increased retention of water and therefore an increased extracellular fluid volume. If for some reason a person has increased resorption of sodium but is unable to take in additional fluid, the concentration of extracellular sodium will increase. Usually the concentration of extracellular sodium does not increase even with increased resorption of sodium, however, because the person drinks more fluid and therefore dilutes the retained sodium.

If a person has an increased resorption of sodium and

increase

is unable to take in additional fluid, the concentration of sodium will _____.

338 Symptoms of hypernatremia are caused by the hypertonicity of the extracellular fluids and the lack of water. Therefore the symptoms will be those of dehydration. The mucous membranes will be dry, the skin flushed, the temperature elevated, and the urine output decreased.

If there is increased resorption of sodium without an increase in fluid intake, the symptoms will be those of

dehydration

_____.

339 Hypernatremia rarely occurs, since usually the fluid intake is increased when sodium is resorbed. The more common problem with sodium excess is an increased extracellular fluid volume that results in edema.

increase

Sodium excess is likely to cause an (increase? decrease?) in extracellular fluid volume.

340 The symptoms will depend on the location of the edema. Edema of the lungs is called *pulmonary* edema and can occur in congestive heart failure. We have considered pulmonary edema previously (frames 260 and 288).

Symptoms of pulmonary edema include the following:

shortness of breath **a** _____

coughing **b** _____

cyanosis **c** _____

increased respiratory rate **d** _____

341 If the edema is in the abdominal cavity, as occurs with congestive heart failure or cirrhosis of the liver, the symptoms will result from the condition causing the ascites and the pressure caused by the fluid. Edema in any tissue will interfere with the nutrition of cells because blood flow is limited to those cells.

decreased

Whenever there is edema, the cells do not have good nutrition, because blood flow is (increased? decreased?) to that part.

342 The treatment of hypernatremia accompanied by increased retention of water is aimed at the physiological mechanisms that produced the excess. For example, in the person with pulmonary edema caused by congestive heart failure, the treatment is aimed at strengthening the contractions of the heart.

The aim of treatment is to improve or correct the condition that caused _____ and _____ retention.

sodium; water

343 Another aspect of treatment is restriction of the intake of sodium. The degree of restriction will vary. For some persons, omitting salt in cooking will be an adequate restriction. For others, avoiding all salts of sodium, such as sodium chloride, sodium lactate, and sodium bicarbonate, may be necessary. There may be any degree of restriction between these two extremes. If salt or sodium is restricted, the nurse should be sure the patient understands the reasons for the restriction. The patient and the family must be taught how to prepare food according to the restrictions. At times the intake of water is also restricted. If water is restricted, a schedule should be worked out so that the water or fluid allowed is spaced over 24 hours.

In treating edema caused by retention of sodium and water, the intake of _____ and _____ may be limited.

sodium; water

344 Treatment may involve the use of diuretics, drugs that prevent the resorption of sodium and water.

Diuretics used to treat increased retention of sodium and water act by _____ of sodium and water in the kidneys.

preventing resorption

345 When diuretics are used, the nurse is responsible for keeping an accurate record of intake, output, and daily weight. This information is useful in avoiding overtreatment. It is possible to produce too great a loss of water and sodium as well as other electrolytes, especially potassium.

When diuretics are used, the nurse should record the following:

intake **a** _____

output

daily weight

b _____

c _____

346 If the increased resorption of sodium and water is caused by the overproduction of aldosterone, an antagonist, spironolactone (Aldactone), may be used.

aldosterone

Spironolactone is an antagonist to _____.

347 The treatment of sodium and water retention will depend on the cause but may include restricting sodium and water intake and the use of diuretics.

restricting

Treatment may include _____ sodium and water intake.

SUMMARY

In a healthy person the kidneys regulate the level of sodium. Certain hormonal or hemodynamic factors may cause the kidneys to be unable to maintain this balance. The conditions in which sodium excess (hypernatremia) may be a problem include renal failure with salt retention, inadequate blood flow to the kidneys (as in congestive heart failure), cirrhosis of the liver, overproduction of aldosterone by the adrenal glands, and treatment with large doses of adrenal corticoids.

Usually, when sodium is retained, water intake and/or resorption occurs. Thus the concentration of extracellular sodium does not increase, but rather there is an increase in extracellular fluid volume. The symptoms of this increase depend on the cause and the location of the edema. Treatment may include restriction of sodium and water intake and the use of diuretics.

REVIEW

aldosterone

1 An increase in the hormone _____ will cause an increased resorption of sodium.

aldosterone

2 Inadequate blood flow to the kidneys will stimulate the production of _____, which will increase the resorption of sodium.

3 When an increased amount of sodium is resorbed, the person is stimulated to _____ water.

take in (drink)

4 When diuretics are used, the nurse should record

intake **a** _____

output **b** _____

daily weight **c** _____

CASE STUDY

Jane Folk

1 Jane Folk, age 79, was admitted to the hospital because of vomiting and diarrhea for several days. The following morning her temperature was 105° F, her heart rate was 150 beats/min, and her respirations were 42/min. When the laboratory results were returned, her serum sodium was 153 mEq/L.

high   This serum sodium level of 153 mEq/L is (high? low?).

2 She has not been vomiting, and she has been given a limited amount of fluid intravenously. With her level of serum sodium, you would expect her to have symptoms

dehydration   of (overhydration? dehydration?).

3 Which of the following signs and symptoms would you expect her to have?

✓ _____ **a** Dry, fissured tongue

✓ _____ **b** Dry, warm skin

_____ **c** Urine output of 2000/24 hr

✓ _____ **d** Thirst

POTASSIUM IMBALANCE

348 Potassium is the major cation in the intracellular fluid. However, the level of potassium inside the cell is difficult to measure, so the balance of potassium must be inferred from its extracellular or serum level. Refer to the diagrams on page 13 to compare the amount of potassium in the serum with that in the cell. Serum potassium tends to rise slightly with increasing age, especially

Table 6. Potassium levels in children

Specimen	Age	Normal value (mEq/L)
Serum/plasma	Newborn	3.7–5.0
	Infant	4.1–5.3
	Child	3.4–4.7

From Behrman, R.E., and Vaughn, V.C.: Nelson textbook of pediatrics, ed. 12, Philadelphia, 1983, W.B. Saunders Co.

in healthy elderly men. (See Table 6 for potassium levels in children.) The normal serum potassium level in older children and adults is 3.5 to 5 mEq/L. The serum level of potassium may or may not be an accurate index of the total body potassium. Since only 5% of total body weight is intravascular fluid and 40% is intracellular fluid, the amount of potassium is relatively small in the intravascular fluid.

a The major cation inside the cell is _____.

b The normal level for serum potassium in older children and adults is _____ mEq/L.

potassium

3.5 to 5

349 One of the functions of potassium is to maintain the volume of fluid within the cell. We established earlier (frame 307) that sodium is important in maintaining cell size. Because sodium is the primary cation outside cells and potassium is the primary cation inside cells, both are significant in controlling the movement of fluid in and out of cells by osmosis.

a The primary cation inside cells is _____.

b The primary cation in the extracellular fluid is _____.

c Both sodium and potassium are essential in controlling the movement of fluid in and out of cells by _____.

potassium

sodium

osmosis

350 Potassium is important in maintaining the volume of fluid within the cell. It is also necessary for the transmission of electrochemical impulses along the membranes of nerve and muscle cells. Therefore potassium is essential in regulating neuromuscular irritability. Potassium easily diffuses through the cell membrane and thus moves positive electrical charges from inside the cell to outside the cell.

a Potassium is (a cation? an anion?).

a cation

b Therefore potassium carries a (positive? negative?) electrical charge.

positive

c Potassium is necessary for the control of electrical impulses in ＿＿＿＿＿＿＿＿ and ＿＿＿＿＿＿＿＿ cells.

nerve; muscle

351 So far we have seen that potassium is important for the control of fluid volume within the cell and for regulating neuromuscular irritability. Another function of potassium is to control the hydrogen ion concentration. When potassium ions move out of the cell, sodium and hydrogen ions move into the cell. The usual ratio is three potassium ions for two sodium and one hydrogen ion (3 K^+ to 2 Na^+ and 1 H^+).

a When one cation moves out of the cell, another ＿＿＿＿＿＿＿＿ moves in to take its place.

cation

b As potassium ions move out of the cell, ＿＿＿＿＿ and ＿＿＿＿＿＿ ions move into the cell.

sodium

hydrogen

c This exchange of cations is usually in the ratio of ＿＿＿＿＿ potassium ions for ＿＿＿＿＿ sodium ions and one hydrogen ion.

three; two

352 Potassium is important in controlling intracellular fluid volume, neuromuscular irritability, and hydrogen ion concentration. The clinical signs and symptoms of potassium imbalance result primarily from altered neuromuscular irritability.

Three functions of potassium are the regulation of

a ＿＿＿＿＿＿＿＿＿＿＿＿＿＿＿＿＿＿＿＿＿＿＿＿＿

intracellular fluid volume

b ＿＿＿＿＿＿＿＿＿＿＿＿＿＿＿＿＿＿＿＿＿＿＿＿＿

neuromuscular irritability

c ＿＿＿＿＿＿＿＿＿＿＿＿＿＿＿＿＿＿＿＿＿＿＿＿＿

H+ concentration

353 Normally potassium is ingested in the diet. Since it is present in many foods, a person who is eating a diet that is adequate in calories and protein will likely have an adequate intake of potassium. Normally a balance in the potassium level is maintained, with 80% to 90% of the potassium being excreted in the urine and the rest being eliminated in the feces and sweat.[18]

a Potassium normally enters the body in the form of ＿＿＿＿＿＿＿＿.

food (diet)

urine

b About 80% to 90% of the potassium intake is excreted in the _____.

354 We are far from having a complete picture of how the concentration of potassium in the body is regulated. Regardless of whether the intake is low, normal, or high, there is a somewhat fixed resorption of filtered potassium in the proximal tubules that is not regulated by any known mechanism.[18] Therefore the filtered potassium is almost totally resorbed.

potassium

Resorption of filtered _____ occurs regardless of intake.

355 Although the filtered potassium is resorbed in the proximal tubules, the regulated excretion of potassium occurs in the distal tubules. The variations in excretion of potassium involve changes in potassium secretion and/ or further potassium resorption.[20] This regulation of potassium excretion is related to several other processes, which include sodium resorption, hydrogen ion excretion, and aldosterone level. For potassium to be excreted, adequate amounts of sodium must be available for exchange. When there is an increase in hydrogen ion excretion, there is a decrease in potassium excretion. An increased level of aldosterone stimulates an increased excretion of potassium.

Which of the following stimulate an increased excretion of potassium?

_____ **a** Sodium deficit

✓   _____ **b** Decreased excretion of hydrogen ions

✓   _____ **c** Increased level of aldosterone

_____ **d** Acidosis

356 When body fluids become too alkaline, the kidneys preserve hydrogen ions and excrete more potassium ions in exchange. Thus, with alkalosis, large amounts of potassium may be excreted in the urine.

more

When alkalosis exists, (more? less?) potassium is excreted in the urine.

357 The feedback mechanism of aldosterone in regulating potassium excretion is exactly opposite that for sodium regulation. When extracellular *sodium* concentration is *low*, aldosterone secretion is increased and more sodium is resorbed. When the extracellular level of *potassium* is *high*, more aldosterone is secreted and more potassium is excreted.

When the production of aldosterone is stimulated, sodium is retained in the body and potassium is _____.

excreted

Potassium deficit

358 We have considered the function of potassium and the mechanisms for its control. We shall now look at the problem of a potassium deficit. Hypopotassemia, called *hypokalemia* (from the Latin word for potassium, "kalium"), is a low serum potassium level. Remember that clinically we cannot measure the intracellular potassium. The serum potassium level may not be an accurate index of the total body potassium level.

A low serum level of potassium is called _____ , or _____.

hypokalemia
hypopotassemia

359 A low serum potassium level may occur when alkalosis is present because potassium moves into the cells. In alkalosis the serum potassium level may be low even though there is not any loss of total body potassium.

In (acidosis? alkalosis?) the serum potassium level may be low even though the total body potassium level is normal.

alkalosis

360 Potassium loss causes a metabolic alkalosis, and the reverse is also true. A metabolic or respiratory alkalosis causes hypokalemia.

Alkalosis causes and can be caused by _____.

hypokalemia

361 When potassium ions are lost from cells, sodium and hydrogen ions move into the cells to replace the potassium. Therefore the hydrogen ion concentration is decreased in the extracellular fluid and metabolic alkalosis results.

Hypokalemia will lead to metabolic (acidosis? alkalosis?).

alkalosis

362 We shall now consider some of the causes of hypokalemia. In general, hypokalemia is caused by either a decreased intake of potassium or an increased loss of potassium.

Hypokalemia may be caused by (increased? decreased?) intake and/or by _____ loss.

decreased
increased

363 Since normal kidneys continue to excrete some potassium, the body must replace it. Normally the intake of potassium is adequate in food and fluids. In a patient who is unable to eat a normal diet, potassium must be given by medication orally or via intravenous fluids. If a patient is given large amounts of intravenous fluids without potassium, hypopotassemia will result.

In a patient who is unable to eat a normal or adequate diet, supplements of potassium (will? will not?) be necessary.

will

364 Even with an adequate intake of potassium, hypokalemia may occur if there is excessive loss of potassium. One way potassium may be lost is through the gastrointestinal tract. Vomiting, gastric suction, intestinal fistulas, or diarrhea can cause a severe potassium loss.

A serious depletion of potassium can occur when gastrointestinal secretions are lost through

vomiting
gastric suction
intestinal fistulas
diarrhea

a _____
b _____
c _____
d _____

365 Hypokalemia may occur through loss of fluids from the gastrointestinal tract. Loss of potassium may also occur through the urinary tract in several conditions. A high sodium intake or excessive administration of bicarbonate or other alkaline substances will stimulate the urinary loss of potassium.

More potassium will be lost in the urine if the intake of sodium is (high? low?).

high

366 Another cause of hypokalemia is certain diseases of the kidneys. Hypokalemia may occur in renal tubular acidosis, in potassium-losing nephritis, and when the patient has had a ureteroenterostomy.

Hypokalemia may occur in certain kidney diseases

increased because of (increased? decreased?) excretion of potassium.

367 Potassium can be lost in the urine as a result of treatment with diuretics. The thiazides and furosemide (Lasix) cause loss of potassium and are more likely to cause hypokalemia in the elderly than in younger adults. While potassium-sparing diuretics (such as triamterene) are more likely to cause *hyper*kalemia in elderly persons than in younger adults, hypokalemia is likely to occur whenever certain diuretics are used, even though they may be necessary in sodium and fluid volume excess.

Use of furosemide or thiazide diuretics may result in
hypo- (hyper-? hypo-?)kalemia.

368 Use of adrenal cortical steroid hormones will increase the excretion of potassium. Earlier (frames 355 and 357) we learned that increased levels of aldosterone will stimulate the excretion of potassium. Therefore overproduction of adrenal cortical hormones or prolonged treatment with steroid drugs will cause loss of potassium.

An increase in adrenal cortical steroid hormones will
increased cause (increased? decreased?) excretion of potassium.

369 We have seen that hypokalemia may be caused by inadequate intake or by increased loss of potassium.

Potassium loss may occur through the gastrointestinal tract with vomiting, gastric suction, intestinal fis-
diarrhea tulas, or _____.

370 Increased amounts of potassium may be lost through the urinary tract in certain kidney diseases, with the use of certain diuretics, or with increased amounts of adrenal cortical steroid hormones (such as cortisone preparations).

Hypokalemia may occur through the increased urinary excretion of potassium caused by

kidney disease **a** _____

certain diuretics **b** _____

adrenal cortical hormones **c** _____

371 The clinical signs and symptoms of hypokalemia are

not specific and may occur in seriously ill patients who do not have low serum potassium.[8] Potassium depletion may be evidenced by neuromuscular signs that include muscular cramps, paresthesias, muscular weakness progressing to flaccid paralysis, fatigue, and mental confusion.

The neuromuscular signs of hypokalemia include

cramps

a paresthesias and muscle _____

flaccid paralysis

b muscular weakness that may progress to _____
_____

confusion

c fatigue and mental (alertness? confusion?)

372 The gastrointestinal signs of hypokalemia result from a reduction of neuromuscular irritability and a weakness of the smooth muscles of the gastrointestinal tract. Therefore a low level of potassium in the body may cause anorexia, abdominal distention, and paralytic ileus (absent peristalsis).

Hypokalemia may cause the following gastrointestinal signs:

anorexia

a _____

abdominal distention

b _____

paralytic ileus

c _____

373 The most important abnormality of renal function when the level of potassium in the body is low is the inability of the kidneys to concentrate urine. Therefore the quantity of urine is increased.

When the level of potassium in the body is low, the output of urine is (increased? unaffected? decreased?).

increased

374 Extreme depletion of potassium involves the respiratory muscles. The diaphragm may be paralyzed. Respirations will become shallow, and death may result from apnea and respiratory arrest.

A severe deficit in potassium will cause (shallow? deep?) respirations.

shallow

375 The cardiac signs of hypokalemia include irregular rhythm, heart block, altered electrocardiograph (ECG) patterns, circulatory failure, hypotension, and systolic arrest.

Hypokalemia may cause cardiac signs that include

irregular **a** (regular? irregular?) rhythm
abnormal **b** (normal? abnormal?) ECG patterns
arrest **c** circulatory failure, hypotension, and systolic _____

376 A deficit in potassium will affect repolarization, which is evident on the ECG. In general, the ECG changes include a shortened and depressed S-T segment, a flattened or inverted T wave, a prolonged Q-T interval, and a U wave that is equal to or higher than the T wave.

flat **a** In hypokalemia the T wave is (flat? peaked?).
lengthened **b** The Q-T interval is (shortened? lengthened?).
present **c** A U wave is (present? absent?).

377 The normal serum potassium level varies from 3.5 to 5 mEq/L. When the serum potassium level is 3 mEq/L or lower, signs of hypokalemia may become evident. We must remember that the serum potassium level does not tell us the total body potassium level.

3.5 **a** Normal serum potassium levels vary between _____
5 and _____ mEq/L.
b Signs of hypokalemia may occur when the serum po-
3 tassium level is _____ mEq/L or lower.

378 If the hypokalemia is severe, laboratory tests will indicate metabolic alkalosis.

alkalosis In severe hypokalemia the laboratory tests will indicate metabolic (acidosis? alkalosis?).

379 A deficit in potassium enhances the action of digitalis. Therefore, if digitalis is given to a person with hypokalemia, digitalis toxicity is more likely to occur.

low A toxic reaction to digitalis is more likely to occur if the potassium is (high? normal? low?).

380 Treatment of hypokalemia is aimed at replacing the potassium that has been lost. Potassium can be given intravenously to achieve a quick response. Potassium given orally is also effective. However, the most natural way to replace potassium is through a high-potassium diet. Many foods contain potassium. Fruit juices (especially orange juice), bananas, bouillon, and meat broths are rich sources.

Foods rich in potassium include

orange juice **a** _____

bananas **b** _____

bouillon **c** _____

meat broths **d** _____

381 If potassium is to be replaced by oral medication, there are several forms that may be used: potassium chloride, potassium citrate, potassium gluconate (Kaon), or combinations of these. Potassium-containing medications must be administered with caution because hyperkalemia can result from excessive dosages. Oliguria is an important sign of toxicity when potassium supplements are given.

decreased

A sign to be watched for when potassium medications are being administered is (increased? decreased?) urinary output.

382 There is no formula for calculating the amount of potassium needed to replace that which is lost, since most of the body's potassium is intracellular. Average deficits are in amounts of 200 to 400 mEq. However, the deficit may be as much as 800 to 1000 mEq of potassium.[8]

200; 1000

The range of deficit may be from _____ to _____ mEq of potassium.

383 If potassium is given intravenously, the rate must be limited. Forty milliequivalents of potassium should be diluted in 1000 ml of intravenous fluid for an adult. When potassium is given intravenously to an adult, the rate of infusion should not exceed 20 mEq/hr.[8] When potassium is given to a child through a peripheral vein, the concentration should not exceed 30 to 40 mEq/L. Potassium supplements for a child are usually calculated at approximately 2 to 4 mEq/kg/24 hr.[12]

a When potassium chloride is given intravenously to an adult, it must be diluted and given at a rate of not more than _____ mEq of potassium per hour.

20

b When potassium is given intravenously to a child, the usual dose is calculated according to the _____ of the child.

weight

384 The reason why potassium-containing solutions

137

should not be given too rapidly intravenously is that the heart muscle is very sensitive to extracellular potassium. If the concentration of potassium rises too rapidly, cardiac arrest may occur. When potassium is administered intravenously, the patient must be observed for symptoms of hyperkalemia. (Hyperkalemia will be discussed later—frames 385 to 401.)

If intravenous potassium is administered too rapidly, death may occur from cardiac _____.

arrest

SUMMARY

Potassium is the major cation in the intracellular fluid. It is necessary to maintain the volume of fluid within the cell, to regulate neuromuscular irritability, and to maintain the hydrogen ion concentration in the body. Normally potassium is ingested with the diet and excreted by the kidneys. Normal kidneys will continue to excrete potassium even with inadequate intake, however, so the regulation of potassium excretion depends on the amount of sodium available for exchange, the number of hydrogen ions being excreted, and the aldosterone level.

Clinically we do not measure the intracellular potassium; therefore the serum potassium level that is measured may not represent accurately the total body potassium. A low serum potassium is associated with alkalosis. Hypokalemia may be caused by a decreased intake or an increased output of potassium.

Depletion of potassium may occur when gastrointestinal secretions are lost through vomiting, gastric suction, intestinal fistulas, or diarrhea. Certain diseases of the kidney, treatment with diuretics, or increased adrenal cortical steroid hormones may also cause hypokalemia.

The clinical signs and symptoms of hypokalemia are not specific but include neuromuscular signs of muscle cramps, paresthesias, muscular weakness progressing to paralysis, fatigue, and mental confusion. The gastrointestinal signs of hypokalemia include anorexia, abdominal distention, and paralytic ileus. The kidneys are unable to concentrate urine. The respirations become shallow, and death may result from apnea and respiratory arrest. The cardiac signs include irregular rhythm, heart block, altered ECG patterns, circulatory failure, hypotension, and systolic arrest. The normal serum potassium level is 3.5 to 5 mEq/L. The treatment of hypokalemia is replacement of the potassium.

REVIEW

potassium

1 The major intracellular cation is _____.

will

2 The kidneys (will? will not?) continue to excrete potassium when the intake of potassium is low.

3 Depletion of potassium may occur when gastrointestinal secretions are lost through any of the following:

vomiting **a** _____

gastric suction **b** _____

intestinal fistulas **c** _____

diarrhea **d** _____

are not

4 Clinical signs and symptoms of hypokalemia (are? are not?) specific.

paralysis

5 One of the symptoms of hypokalemia is muscular weakness that may progress to _____.

3.5 to 5

6 The normal serum potassium level is _____ mEq/L.

is not

7 The serum potassium level (is? is not?) always an accurate picture of the total body potassium level.

8 Which of the following will have a greater loss of potassium?

✓ _____ **a** A person taking a diuretic

_____ **b** A person taking a laxative

Potassium excess

385 Since normally functioning kidneys excrete potassium, abnormal accumulation of potassium in the body

139

does not occur often. However, hyperpotassemia (or hyperkalemia) can occur and is extremely dangerous. One cause of hyperkalemia is excessive parenteral administration of potassium or overly rapid administration of solutions containing potassium.

does not occur

a Hyperkalemia (occurs? does not occur?) frequently.

hyper-

b Excessive parenteral administration of potassium can cause (hyper-? hypo-?)kalemia.

386 Trauma to tissues (such as crush injuries) will liberate intracellular potassium and result in hyperkalemia.

Intracellular potassium may be liberated by tissue

crush

trauma such as occurs in _____ injuries.

387 Adrenal cortical insufficiency will cause hyperkalemia. For example, in Addison's disease, in which aldosterone is lacking, potassium is not excreted normally. Therefore the level of potassium in the body goes up.

insufficiency

Adrenal cortical (insufficiency? overactivity?) will cause hyperkalemia.

388 Respiratory or metabolic acidosis may cause the serum potassium level to rise. In acidosis the hydrogen ion concentration in the extracellular fluid increases. This causes potassium to move out of the cells; then hydrogen and sodium ions move into the cell. Therefore the level of potassium in the serum increases.

hyper-

a Acidosis may cause (hypo-? hyper-?)kalemia.

hypo-

b Alkalosis may cause (hypo-? hyper-?)kalemia.

389 In a patient with renal failure, the serum level of potassium may be difficult to control. Hyperkalemia is more likely to occur after the urinary output falls below 400 to 500 ml/day.[8]

hyper-

In renal failure with a decreased urinary output, (hyper-? hypo-?)kalemia may occur.

390 Some of the more common causes of hyperkalemia include excessive administration of potassium, tissue trauma that liberates intracellular potassium, adrenal cortical insufficiency, acidosis, and renal failure with decreased urinary output. The major danger of hyperkalemia is its effect on the myocardium.

The danger of hyperkalemia is the effect on the _____.

heart (myocardium)

391 Hyperkalemia is a medical emergency because of its effect on the heart. The danger is that the patient will die of cardiac standstill. When the extracellular potassium is elevated to 7 mEq/L or more, heart block and ventricular standstill may occur.[18] When complete heart block is associated with hyperkalemia, the rate may be slow and the heart is in danger of stopping in diastole.

3.5 to 5

a Normal serum potassium is _____ mEq/L.

7

b Heart block or ventricular standstill may occur when the serum potassium is elevated to _____ mEq/L or more.

392 Neuromuscular symptoms of hyperkalemia include weakness that may progress to flaccid paralysis. Respiratory paralysis and involvement of the muscles of phonation may occur. Both hypokalemia and severe hyperkalemia may cause muscle paralysis. Movement of potassium and sodium is necessary for polarization and the spread of stimuli along the muscle fibers. If either persistent increased or decreased polarizaton occurs, the spread of the stimuli is blocked along the muscle fibers and muscle weakness or paralysis follows.

both hypo- and hyper-

Muscle weakness or paralysis is a symptom of (hypo-? hyper-? both hypo- and hyper-?)kalemia.

393 Both hypokalemia and hyperkalemia may cause muscle weakness and paralysis. Paresthesias, or numbness and tingling sensations, are common in hyperkalemia. Paresthesias caused by hyperkalemia usually affect the face, tongue, hands, and feet.[8]

hyper-

Paresthesias of the face, tongue, hands, and feet may be the result of (hypo-? hyper-?)kalemia.

394 The ECG changes in hyperkalemia include tall peaked T waves, widening of the QRS complex, and shortening of the Q-T interval. This is just the reverse of the ECG changes that occur in hypokalemia. Later the P-R interval becomes prolonged, and then the P waves flatten or disappear.

ECG changes that occur in hyperkalemia include the following:

a T waves are _____.

b Q-T interval is (shortened? lengthened?).

c The _____ wave disappears.

395 The laboratory findings in hyperkalemia include a serum potassium of 6 mEq/L or higher.

a The normal serum potassium level is _____ mEq/L.

b Serum potassium levels of _____ mEq/L or higher are present in hyperkalemia.

396 Other laboratory findings would be respiratory or metabolic acidosis. Hyperkalemia occurs in both respiratory and metabolic acidosis and is probably a compensatory mechanism. In acidosis the hydrogen ion concentration of the extracellular fluid increases. The potassium ions move out of the cells and into the extracellular fluid, and hydrogen and sodium ions move into the cells.[8]

In hyperkalemia laboratory findings of respiratory or metabolic (acidosis? alkalosis?) may be present.

397 The aim of treatment is to find the cause and correct it when possible. The method used to treat hyperkalemia will depend on the cause and severity of the hyperkalemia and on the patient's homeostatic mechanisms. An uncomplicated excess of potassium can be treated by avoiding additional potassium intake either orally or parenterally. A serum potassium level of 6.5 mEq/L and an abnormal ECG are considered an emergency. The immediate treatment is aimed at inducing potassium to enter the cells. Hypertonic glucose may be given intravenously to help potassium shift from the extracellular fluid to the liver and muscle cells.

a A serum potassium level of _____ mEq/L with an abnormal ECG is considered an emergency.

b Hypertonic glucose is given to help potassium move (into? out of?) cells.

398 Insulin is given with the glucose to induce the movement of potassium back into the cells. Sodium bicarbonate may be used to buffer the hydrogen ion and allow the potassium to return to the cells.

The use of glucose, insulin, and sodium bicarbonate
move into the cell · is aimed at helping the potassium to _____
_____.

399 Calcium gluconate may be administered intravenously in the treatment of hyperkalemia to increase the
movement of potassium ions into tissue cells. Testosterone may be administered to prevent excessive protein
breakdown and facilitate diffusion of potassium into bone
and tissue cells.

Both calcium gluconate and testosterone are useful
in making possible the movement of potassium from the
cells · extracellular fluid into the _____.

400 Drugs such as cation-exchange resins may be used
to remove potassium from the body through the gastrointestinal tract. The cation-exchange resin, which is of the
carboxylic acid type, gives up hydrogen ions for cations
(e.g., potassium, sodium, calcium). The resin can be
given orally or rectally. The resins may cause constipation
or impaction, and a mild laxative may be necessary.

Cation-exchange resins may be used in the treatment
of hyperkalemia and act to remove potassium by way of
gastrointestinal · the _____ tract.

401 If these measures are not successful in lowering the
serum potassium level, or if there is renal failure, the
hyperkalemia should be treated by peritoneal dialysis or
hemodialysis.

Hyperkalemia caused by renal failure should be treat-
peritoneal dialysis or · ed by _____.
hemodialysis

SUMMARY

Hyperkalemia does not occur often, since normal kidneys continue to excrete potassium even when the intake
is not adequate. However, when it does occur, it may be
caused by excessive parenteral administration of potassium, crush injuries, adrenal cortical insufficiency, and
respiratory or metabolic acidosis. Another possible cause
is renal failure with oliguria (decreased urinary output).

143

The signs and symptoms of hyperkalemia are similar to those of hypokalemia except for the greater effect of hyperkalemia on the heart muscle.

Heart block and ventricular standstill may occur if the extracellular potassium is 7 mEq/L or more. Muscle weakness and paralysis are symptoms of both hypokalemia and hyperkalemia. Paresthesias caused by hyperkalemia usually affect the face, tongue, hands, and feet.

In hyperkalemia the ECG changes include tall peaked T waves, widening of the QRS complex, and a shortened Q-T interval. The P-R interval becomes prolonged, and then the P waves flatten or disappear. A serum potassium level of 6 mEq/L or more is present in hyperkalemia. The immediate treatment is aimed at inducing potassium to enter the cells.

REVIEW

Hyperkalemia

1 _____ may be caused by excessive administration of potassium.

insufficiency

2 Crush injuries and adrenal cortical (insufficiency? overactivity?) may cause hyperkalemia.

acidosis

3 Hyperkalemia may be caused by respiratory or metabolic (acidosis? alkalosis?).

low

4 In a person with renal failure, hyperkalemia is more likely to occur when the urinary output is (high? low?).

6

5 A serum potassium level of _____ mEq/L or more is present in hyperkalemia.

CASE STUDY
Cindy Jackson

1 Cindy Jackson has been admitted to the hospital complaining of increasing weakness. Ms. Jackson has multiple sclerosis, but she has been living alone and had been getting from her bed into her wheelchair by herself. Recently, she has been unable to even turn over in bed.

When her electrolyte report comes from the laboratory, you find the following: sodium, 139 mEq/L; potassium, 1 mEq/L; chloride, 96 mEq/L.

a Which of the electrolytes is the most abnormal?

potassium
_____

b With a very low potassium you would expect to find

weakness
muscular _____ .

c The most likely cause for Ms. Jackson's inability to

low potassium
turn over in bed is (exacerbation of her multiple sclerosis? low potassium?).

2 In further discussion with Ms. Jackson, you learn that her feet had been swelling and the physician had given her Lasix (diuretic) pills to take one per day. Recently the swelling has not gone down overnight, so she has been taking several extra Lasix tablets to reduce the swelling.

The explanation for Ms. Jackson's weakness is the

excretion
low potassium caused by urinary (excretion? retention?) due to the Lasix without adequate intake of potassium.

MAGNESIUM IMBALANCE

402 Magnesium is the fourth most abundant cation in the body. Like potassium, most of the magnesium is intracellular. Therefore only small amounts of magnesium are present in the serum. Refer to the diagrams on page 13 to compare the amount of magnesium in the intracellular compartment with that in the intravascular and the interstitial compartments.

intracellular
a Most of the magnesium in the body is in the (intravascular? intracellular? interstitial?) compartment.

interstitial
b The smallest amount of magnesium is in the (intravascular? intracellular? interstitial?) compartment.

403 Approximately 50% of the total magnesium content of the body is present in bone. Only about 1% of the body's magnesium is in the extracellular fluid. The normal serum level of magnesium is 1.5 to 2.5 mEq/L.

a The percent of magnesium that is extracellular is

1
_____ .

1.5; 2.5
b The normal serum magnesium is _____ to _____ mEq/L.

145

404 Magnesium has several essential functions. The importance of magnesium has been recognized more recently than that of some other electrolytes. Magnesium functions as an activator in many enzyme reactions. Some of the enzyme systems that magnesium activates are those that empower the B vitamins to function and those that are associated with carbohydrate and protein metabolism. Magnesium is required for the synthesis of nucleic acids and proteins.

a Magnesium is necessary as an activator of many

_____ systems.

b The synthesis of nucleic acid and proteins requires

_____.

405 Another function of magnesium is that it exerts an effect similar to that of calcium on neuromuscular function. At some points magnesium acts synergistically with calcium, while at others it is antagonistic. Magnesium affects skeletal muscle directly by depressing acetylcholine release at the synaptic junction. Therefore neuromuscular activity is increased when magnesium levels are decreased. Magnesium is commonly used to prevent convulsions in eclampsia (toxemia) of pregnancy.

When magnesium levels are increased, neuromuscular activity is (increased? decreased?).

406 So far we have seen that magnesium is essential as an activator in many enzyme reactions. It is especially necessary for carbohydrate metabolism, and it is required for the synthesis of nucleic acids and proteins. Magnesium affects neuromuscular functions; it also facilitates the transportation of sodium and potassium across cell membranes. If magnesium is deficient, the kidneys tend to excrete more potassium.

When magnesium is deficient, the kidneys are likely to excrete (more? less?) potassium.

407 Magnesium also influences the levels of intracellular calcium through its effect on parathyroid hormone secretions. If the level of magnesium in the body is below normal, the action of parathyroid hormone in maintaining normal serum calcium levels is impaired.

Magnesium influences the level of intracellular calcium by its effect on the secretion of _____ _____.

408 Magnesium therefore functions as an activator in many enzyme reactions, in carbohydrate and protein metabolism, in the synthesis of nucleic acids and proteins, in neuromuscular function, and in the transportation of sodium and potassium across cell membranes, and it influences the levels of intracellular calcium. A healthy adult ingests about 25 mEq (180 to 300 mg) of magnesium per day, while a child requires 150 to 250 mg of magnesium per day. A major source of dietary magnesium is the chlorophyll in green vegetables.

a A major source of dietary magnesium is _____ _____.

b A healthy adult ingests approximately _____ mEq of magnesium per day.

409 While a major source of magnesium is green vegetables, other foods also contain magnesium. It is abundant in nuts, legumes, and fruit such as bananas, grapefruit, and oranges. Magnesium is also plentiful in peanut butter and chocolate.

Which of the following foods contain abundant amounts of magnesium?

_____ **a** Green beans
_____ **b** Milk
_____ **c** Walnuts
_____ **d** Honey
_____ **e** Peanut butter

410 Magnesium is absorbed from the intestine. A number of physiological factors influence normal absorption, including the total magnesium intake; the length of time it is in the intestine; the rate of water absorption; and the amounts of calcium, phosphate, and lactose in the diet. It is therefore understandable that persons who have had intestinal bypass surgery for obesity may develop magnesium deficiency.

a Magnesium is usually taken into the body in the normal _____.

b Magnesium is absorbed from the _____.

411 Magnesium is lost from the body primarily in the urine. The kidneys are able to conserve magnesium ions, so that renal excretion may be less than 1 mEq/day on a magnesium-free diet, after a period of adjustment.

in the urine

a The major pathway for magnesium loss is _____ _____.

are

b The kidneys (are? are not?) able to conserve magnesium.

Magnesium deficit (hypomagnesemia)

412 We have considered the function, as well as the intake and loss, of magnesium. Most of the factors that control magnesium metabolism are not known.[8] The major site of regulation is probably intracellular, but its mechanism is unknown.[18] A low serum magnesium level is called hypomagnesemia. Hypomagnesemia is present when the serum concentration of magnesium is less than 1.5 mEq/L.

1.5; 2.5

a Normal serum magnesium is _____to _____ mEq/L.

1.5

b Hypomagnesemia is present when the serum magnesium is less than _____ mEq/L.

413 Remember that only 1% of the magnesium in the body is extracellular. Therefore there is no direct correlation between serum concentration and the total body stores of magnesium. Usually when symptoms are present, the serum magnesium concentraton will be below 1 mEq/L.

When symptoms of hypomagnesemia are present, the serum magnesium usually will be below _____ mEq/L.

1

414 A deficit in magnesium is not usually a result of dietary restrictions. However, it can occur with prolonged malnutrition or starvation, or if a patient is given magnesium-free fluids intravenously along with no oral intake and/or with nasogastric suction. Persons receiving parenteral hyperalimentation (total parenteral nutrition) in which there is inadequate magnesium may develop hypomagnesemia.

a An inadequate intake of magnesium will lead to

hypomagnesemia

_____.

do

b Persons who are receiving no oral intake (do? do not?) need magnesium added to the intravenous fluids.

415 Hypomagnesemia can be caused by inadequate intake, as discussed in frame 414. A more common cause is impaired intestinal absorption.

Impaired intestinal absorption of magnesium will lead

hypomagnesemia

to _____.

416 Children or adults with malabsorption syndrome (nontropical sprue or steatorrhea) or chronic diarrhea may develop hypomagnesemia. Persons with gastrointestinal fistulas may also develop hypomagnesemia. In these persons magnesium is excreted in the stool in the form of magnesium soaps.

Persons with malabsorption syndrome or chronic diar-

hypo-

rhea may develop (hyper-? hypo-?) magnesemia.

417 Another cause of hypomagnesemia is an excessive intake of calcium, which impairs magnesium absorption, since they compete for the same absorption site.

Hypomagnesemia may be caused by an excessive in-

calcium

take of _____.

418 Magnesium deficit can be induced by alcoholism. Alcohol ingestion seems to promote a magnesium deficit that is unrelated to dietary intake.[31]

Alcohol ingestion seems to promote a magnesium

deficit

(deficit? excess?).

419 Other causes of impaired absortion of magnesium include bowel resection, small bowel bypass, or inherited intestinal defects in magnesium absorption.

Bowel resection may contribute to a magnesium

deficit

(deficit? excess?).

420 We have considered inadequate intake of magnesium and impaired absorption as causes of hypomagnesemia. Other causes of hypomagnesemia include excessive renal excretion or fluid loss.

Three categories of causes of hypomagnesemia include

inadequate intake   **a** _____

impaired absorption   **b** _____

excessive loss   **c** _____

421 The usual cause of excessive renal excretion of magnesium is diuretic therapy. Hypomagnesemia may be clinically significant when produced by diuretic therapy because many of these persons are also taking digitalis. There is evidence that digitalis toxicity can be aggravated by hypomagnesemia.

diuretic

A common cause of excessive renal excretion of magnesium is _____ therapy.

422 Another cause of hypomagnesemia is major surgery. Following major surgery, excessive urinary loss of magnesium occurs for 24 hours.

loss

During the first 24 hours following major surgery, excessive urinary (loss? retention?) of magnesium occurs.

423 Increased magnesium loss also occurs in diabetic ketoacidosis, primary aldosteronism, primary hyperparathyroidism, and other hypercalcemic states.

increased

In diabetic ketoacidosis (increased? decreased?) magnesium loss occurs.

424 Excessive urinary excretion of magnesium may occur with several types of renal disease.

magnesium

Renal disease may cause increased urinary excretion of _____.

425 In considering excessive renal loss of magnesium we have included diuretic therapy, major surgery, diabetic ketoacidosis, primary aldosteronism, primary hyperparathyroidism, and other hypercalcemic states as well as renal disease. Hypomagnesemia may also occur in hypoparathyroidism in association with hypocalcemia. Whenever hypocalcemia and hypokalemia exist, expect to find hypomagnesemia.

low

When a person has a low calcium and a low potassium level, you should expect to find a (high? low?) level of magnesium.

426 We have seen that hypomagnesemia may be caused by inadequate intake, impaired absorption, or excessive renal excreton. While the clinical picture varies from patient to patient, certain signs and symptoms are frequently seen. Remember that one of the actions of magnesium is its effect on neuromuscular function. The signs and symptoms of magnesium deficit are characterized by neuromuscular irritability; these include tremor, athetoid or choreiform movements, tetany, increased reflexes, clonus, a positive Babinski's sign, a positive Chvostek's sign, paresthesias of the feet and legs, excessive neuromuscular irritability, and convulsions.

A positive Babinski's sign is the dorsiflexion of the great toe with fanning of the other toes when the lateral aspect of the sole is stroked sharply. However, in an infant this is a normal response up until about age 2 years. Chvostek's sign is elicited by tapping the person's face just in front of the ear over the facial nerve. Tapping over the nerve will cause unilateral spasm of the lip, nose, or eyelid when the test is positive.

Babinski's reflex. 1, Direction of stroke. 2, Dorsiflexion of big toe. 3, Fanning of toes. (From Whaley, L.F., and Wong, D.L.: Nursing care of infants and children, ed. 3, St. Louis, 1987, The C.V. Mosby Co.)

irritability

a The signs and symptoms of magnesium deficit are characterized by neuromuscular _____.

b Which of the following are signs or symptoms of magnesium deficit?

✔ _____ (1) Tremor

_____ (2) Negative Babinski's sign

✔ _____ (3) Tetany

✔ _____ (4) Increased reflexes

_____ (5) Lethargy

✔ _____ (6) Convulsions

427 Other signs and symptoms of magnesium deficit include personality changes with agitation, mental depression or confusion, and hallucinations, which are usually auditory or visual.

deficit

A person who develops a personality change with agitation or becomes mentally depressed or confused or develops hallucinations may have a magnesium (deficit? excess?).

428 There may be cardiovascular signs of a magnesium deficit, including tachycardia with atrial or ventricular premature contractions, hypotension caused by vasodilation, and nonspecific T wave changes in the electrocardiogram.

Which of the following signs may result from magnesium deficit?

_____ **a** Bradycardia

✔ _____ **b** Atrial or ventricular premature contractions

✔ _____ **c** Hypotension

✔ _____ **d** Nonspecific T wave changes

429 Most of the signs and symptoms of a magnesium deficit are related to the neuromuscular, neurological, or cardiovascular systems. Hypomagnesemia and hypocalcemia may coexist. This is especially true in persons with an excessive loss of gastrointestinal fluids.

a Most of the signs and symptoms of a magnesium

neurological
neuromuscular
cardiovascular

deficit are related to the _____, _____, and _____ systems.

hypo-

b When hypocalcemia is present, (hyper-? hypo-?)magnesemia may also be present.

430 Hypomagnesemia and hypercalcemia may also co-exist in hyperparathyroid persons and in persons who have neoplastic disease with osteolytic metastasis (metastasis to bone).

In persons with hyperparathyroid function or who have neoplastic disease with metastasis to bone, hypomagnesemia may coexist with (hypo-? hyper-?)calcemia.

hyper-

431 A deficit in magnesium may precipitate or aggravate digitalis toxicity.

A toxic reaction to digitalis is more likely to occur if the serum magnesium is (high? low?).

low

432 Treatment of hypomagnesemia consists of correcting the underlying cause of the low serum magnesium. Hypomagnesemia can be treated with magnesium salts intravenously, intramuscularly, or orally. Magnesium sulfate is the most commonly used magnesium salt.

correcting the cause

a Hypomagnesemia should be treated by first _____
_____.

magnesium sulfate

b The most commonly used magnesium salt is _____
_____.

433 Magnesium salts can be given orally to counteract continuous excessive losses. When magnesium is given orally, diarrhea is a possible side effect.

A possible side effect of magnesium salts given orally

diarrhea

is _____.

434 In an adult magnesium sulfate can be given intramuscularly in a dose of 2 g (16.3 mEq) every 8 hours for 3 to 5 days. Repeated intramuscular injections should be given at different sites because the injections may be painful. Procaine hydrochloride 1% can be added to the injection if a large dose is used.

Intramuscular injections of magnesium sulfate are

likely

(likely? not likely?) to be painful.

435 In an adult magnesium sulfate can also be given intravenously when hypomagnesemia is severe and may be associated with convulsions. In an adult, when magnesium is given intravenously, it must not exceed a rate of 150 mg/min. A rate of 1.5 ml/min of a 10% solution

From Perry, A.G., and Potter, P.A.: Clinical nursing skills techniques, St. Louis, 1986, The C.V. Mosby Co.

or 3 ml/min of a 5% solution should not be exceeded an adult.

a The maximum safe rate for giving magnesium in venously in an adult is _____ mg/min.

150

b If you are giving a 10% solution of magnesium, maximum safe rate is _____ ml/min for an adult.

1.5

436 During an intravenous infusion of magnesium s fate, the patient should not be left alone. You sho observe the effectiveness of the magnesium infusion relieving signs and symptoms. Observe for the antic vulsant effect, relaxation of spastic muscles, and re lution of tremors and arrhythmias.

Signs indicating that the magnesium infusion is fective include a decrease in

muscle tension	**a** _____
tremors	**b** _____
arrhythmias	**c** _____

437 Whenever magnesium sulfate is given intravenously, you must monitor the patient for signs and symptoms of high serum magnesium (see frame 452). Check every 5 minutes or prior to each dose for flaccidity and loss of patellar (knee-jerk) reflex.

high

a When giving magnesium sulfate intravenously, you must monitor the patient for signs of (high? low?) serum magnesium.

5

b You should check for loss of the patellar reflex every _____ minutes.

438 In addition to checking for loss of the patellar reflex, you should also count the respiratory rate every 5 minutes. Be sure the respiratory rate is at least 16/min. Respiratory paralysis may occur during infusion of magnesium sulfate.

loss of patellar reflex
respiratory rate

During intravenous infusion of magnesium sulfate, you should check for _____ and _____ every 5 minutes.

439 During intravenous infusion of magnesium sulfate, you should look for flushing of the skin, especially of the face, and for diaphoresis.

redness
moist

Observations to be made during an intravenous infusion of magnesium sulfate include (redness? paleness?) of the face and (moist? dry?) skin.

440 In addition to checking reflexes, respiratory rate, and condition of the skin, you need to check the blood pressure of the person receiving magnesium sulfate intravenously. During an infusion, you should check the patient's blood pressure every 5 to 10 minutes to detect hypotension.

5; 10

During infusion of magnesium sulfate, the blood pressure should be checked every ____ to ____ minutes.

441 When giving intravenous infusion of magnesium sulfate, you should slow or stop the infusion and notify

155

From Perry, A.G., and Potter, P.A.: Clinical nursing skills and techniques, St. Louis, 1986, The C.V. Mosby Co.

the physician if any one of the following signs appears: loss of the patellar reflex, decreased respiratory rate, flushing of the face, diaphoresis, flaccidity, or hypotension.

During intravenous infusion of magnesium sulfate, you should slow or stop the infusion if which of the following signs appear?

✓   _____ **a** Loss of the patellar reflex

     _____ **b** Increased respiratory rate of 24

✓   _____ **c** Flushing of the face

     _____ **d** Spasticity

✓   _____ **e** Hypotension

442 If magnesium levels become high, respiratory failure may occur (see frames 451 through 453).

If magnesium levels become high, you must be prepared to manage respiratory _____.

failure

443 One of the prime responsibilties of the nurse in caring for a person with a magnesium deficit is to provide for the patient's safety. Since convulsions may occur, protective measures must be taken to prevent injury.

Persons with a magnesium deficit must be protected from injury that could result during a _____.

convulsion

444 Another reason why persons with a magnesium deficit have special safety needs is that they may become confused and/or may develop hallucinatons.

Persons with a magnesium deficit need to be protected, since they may become (drowsy? confused?) and may develop hallucinations.

confused

SUMMARY

Magnesium is the second most abundant cation in the intracellular fluid. Magnesium is essential as an activator in many enzyme reactions, especially carbohydrate metabolism. It is required for the synthesis of nucleic acids and proteins, and it is important for normal neuromuscular function. It influences the levels of intracellular calcium and facilitates transportation of sodium and potassium across cell membranes.

Most of the magnesium is in the intracellular fluid. Only about 1% of magnesium is extracellular. Normal serum magnesium is 1.5 to 2.5 mEq/L.

Magnesium deficit may occur with prolonged malnutrition, starvation, alcoholism, or administration of magnesium-free intravenous fluids along with no oral intake. A deficit in magnesium may be caused by impaired intestinal absorption or loss through diarrhea or draining gastrointestinal fistulas. Excessive loss of magnesium may occur through renal excretion.

The clinical signs and symptoms of hypomagnesemia are not specific but may include mental changes such as personality change, agitation, mental depression, confusion, or hallucinations. The neuromuscular signs and symptoms include tremor, tetany, clonus, increased reflexes, positive Babinski's sign, positive Chvostek's sign, paresthesias, and convulsions. The cardiovascular signs and symptoms include tachycardia, atrial or ventricular premature contractions, hypotension, and nonspecific T wave changes in the electrocardiogram.

REVIEW

magnesium

1 The second major intracellular cation is _____.

enzyme

2 Magnesium is essential as an activator in many _____ reactions.

1.5; 2.5

3 Normal serum magnesium is ____ to ____ mEq/L.

4 A magnesium deficit may result from inadequate intake such as

malnutrition or starvation

a _____

alcoholism

b _____

magnesium-free intravenous
fluids

c _____

5 Excessive loss of magnesium may be caused by intestinal conditions such as

malabsorption

a _____

diarrhea

b _____

fistulas

c _____

are not

6 Clinical signs and symptoms of hypomagnesemia (are? are not?) specific.

hypo-

7 Personality change, confusion, or hallucinations may occur with (hypo-? hyper-?)magnesemia.

8 Which of the following are neuromuscular signs and symptoms of hypomagnesemia?

✓

_____ **a** Tremor

_____ **b** Depressed reflexes

✓

_____ **c** Positive Babinski's sign

✓

_____ **d** Convulsions

Magnesium excess

445 Magnesium excess, or hypermagnesemia, is not a common imbalance. Hypermagnesemia seldom develops except in renal failure.

The most common cause of hypermagnesemia is

renal failure

_____.

446 Hypermagnesemia is a serum magnesium level over 2.5 mEq/L.

1.5; 2.5

a Normal serum magnesium is _____ to _____mEq/L.

b A serum magnesium level of 3 mEq/L would be called

hypermagnesemia

_____.

447 While renal failure is the most common cause of hypermagnesemia, excessive use of magnesium-containing medications can also contribute to hypermagnesemia. A person with renal failure who takes large amounts of magnesium-containing antacids or cathartics may develop hypermagnesemia.

A person who takes large amounts of magnesium-containing antacids may develop (hyper-? hypo-?)magnesemia.

hyper-

448 Hypermagnesemia may occur in a person who has diabetic ketoacidosis when there has been severe water loss.

A person who has diabetic ketoacidosis with severe dehydration may develop _____.

hypermagnesemia

449 The signs and symptoms of hypermagnesemia will vary with the level of serum magnesium. When the serum magnesium is between 3 and 5 mEq/L, the vasodilating effect of magnesium can cause hypotension. Flushing, a feeling of warmth, and diaphoresis may also occur.

A patient with a serum magnesium of _____ to _____ mEq/L may have hypotension.

3; 5

450 When the serum magnesium increases to a level of 5 to 7 mEq/L, the person becomes drowsy. At a serum magnesium level of 7 mEq/L, the deep tendon reflexes are lost.[8]

a A person may become drowsy when the serum magnesium is over _____ mEq/L.

5

b When the serum magnesium level is 7 mEq/L, the deep tendon reflexes are (increased? decreased? absent?).

absent

451 The respiratory center is depressed when the serum magnesium rises to 10 mEq/L.[8]

Respiratory depression occurs at a serum level of _____ mEq/L.

10

452 Coma may occur at serum magnesium levels of 12 to 15 mEq/L, and cardiac arrest is likely at concentrations of 15 to 20 mEq/L.[8]

At serum magnesium levels over 15 mEq/L, coma is likely to occur, followed by _____ arrest.

cardiac

453 The sequence of the signs and symptoms of increasing magnesemia are hypotension, drowsiness, loss of deep tendon reflexes, respiratory depression, coma, and cardiac arrest.

Loss of deep tendon reflexes is likely to occur at a serum magnesium level of _____ mEq/L.

7

454 Intervention is aimed at treating the cause of the magnesium excess. Magnesium salts should not be given to persons with renal failure. If renal failure is present, dialysis will likely be necessary even though dialysis is not very efficient in removing magnesium.

Persons with renal failure (should? should not?) take medications containing magnesium salts.

should not

455 Another useful treatment for hypermagnesemia is the use of intravenous calcium gluconate. Calcium has an antagonistic effect on magnesium and can therefore be a useful temporary measure. (See frame 500 for calcium infusions.)

An electrolyte that has an antagonistic effect on magnesium and may be used in treating hypermagnesemia is _____.

calcium

456 The nurse must assess patients for signs and symptoms that would indicate possible increasing hypermagnesemia.

The first step in the nursing care of patients with potential hypermagnesemia is _____.

assessment

SUMMARY

Hypermagnesemia seldom occurs except in persons with renal failure. A serum level of magnesium over 2.5 mEq/L is hypermagnesemia. Excessive use of magnesium-containing medications by a person with renal failure can contribute to hypermagnesemia. Persons with diabetic ketoacidosis and severe water loss may develop hypermagnesemia. The progression of signs and symptoms of hypermagnesemia is from hypotension, flushing, diaphoresis, drowsiness, loss of deep tendon reflexes, and respiratory depression to coma and cardiac arrest.

1 A serum magnesium of 3 mEq/L is ———————.

2 The most common cause of hypermagnesemia is

renal failure ———————————.

3 One of the earliest signs of hypermagnesemia is

hypotension ———————————.

4 At a serum magnesium level of 7 mEq/L, deep tendon

absent reflexes are likely to be ———————.

5 Calcium gluconate is sometimes used in treating hy-

antagonistic permagnesemia because calcium is ——————— to magnesium.

CALCIUM IMBALANCE

457 Serum calcium imbalance can be a real medical emergency; therefore it is important for you to know how the body normally balances calcium and how to anticipate and recognize a calcium imbalance. Calcium is the most abundant cation in the body. However, 99% of the calcium is in the bones.

cation   Calcium is the most abundant (cation? anion?) in the body.

458 The other 1% of the calcium in the body is in the blood plasma or serum. The calcium concentration in the extracellular compartment normally remains remarkably constant. Normally the total serum calcium is in the range of 4.5 to 5.3 mEq/L or 9 to 10.6 mg/100 ml.

1   **a** The amount of calcium in the serum is ——— %.

remains constant   **b** Normally the serum calcium concentration (remains constant? fluctuates widely?).

4.5 to 5.3   **c** The normal serum calcium concentration is (1.5 to 2.5? 3.5 to 5.0? 4.5 to 5.3?) mEq/L.

459 The calcium in the intravascular compartment is mainly in two forms: one form is ionized calcium, which is physiologically active; the second form is the calcium that is bound to protein.

ionized

a The form of calcium that is physiologically active is _____ calcium.

protein

b The bound calcium in the blood is bound to _____.

460 Normally 50% to 75% of the serum calcium is ionized.

active

a Ionized serum calcium is physiologically (inactive? active?).

50; 75

b The amount of serum calcium that is ionized is _____ % to _____ %.

461 While 50% to 75% of the serum calcium is ionized, the rest is bound to protein. Most of the bound calcium is combined with albumin. The calcium that is bound to plasma protein cannot pass through the capillary wall and therefore cannot leave the intravascular compartment.

albumin

a Most of the calcium that is bound to protein is bound to _____.

cannot

b Calcium that is bound to plasma protein (can? cannot?) pass through the capillary wall.

462 Clinically the serum calcium level can be misleading unless it is correlated with the serum albumin level. As the total protein in the blood decreases, less serum calcium is bound.

albumin

a The serum calcium level should be correlated with the serum _____ level.

less

b When the total protein in the blood decreases, (more? less?) calcium is bound.

463 Any change in serum protein will result in a change in the total serum calcium. The amount of that change is about 0.8 mg/100 ml of serum calcium for each 1 g/100 ml of serum protein.

a decrease

A decrease in serum protein will result in (a decrease? an increase?) in serum calcium.

464 One of the functions of calcium, along with phosphorus, is to provide strength and durability to bones and teeth. As we learned earlier, 99% of the calcium is in the bones. While the serum calcium is a small percentage of the total, it is essential for some vital physiological processes.

strength; durability

a Calcium provides _____ and _____ to bones and teeth.

essential

b The calcium in the serum is (essential? nonessential?) for some of the vital physiological processes.

465 Free, ionized calcium is needed to help maintain the permeability of cell membranes. Calcium is essential for the transmission of nerve impulses and neuromuscular excitability, and it is necessary for normal cardiac function.

permeability

a Calcium is necessary to help maintain the _____ of cell membranes.

transmission

b Calcium is necessary for the _____ of nerve impulses.

466 In addition to helping maintain the permeability of cell membranes and influencing neuromuscular function, calcium is needed for blood coagulation.

needed

Calcium is (needed? not needed?) for blood coagulation.

467 Calcium is also important in activating enzyme reactions and hormone secretion.

activating

Calcium functions by _____ enzyme reactions.

468 Within the range that is compatible with life, fluctuations in the concentration of calcium greatly affect the excitability of nerve tissue. Nerve cell membranes are less excitable when sufficient calcium is available.

sedative

Calcium acts as a (sedative? stimulant?) on nerve cell membranes.

469 We have considered some of the functions of calcium. We will now look at the absorption of calcium. Our bodies have an exquisite control system for maintaining the level of calcium in the serum. The serum calcium comes from the resorption of bone, intestinal absorption, and renal tubular resorption.

List three sources of serum calcium:

bone resorption   **a** _____

intestinal absorption   **b** _____

renal resorption   **c** _____

470 Serum calcium is lost by bone deposition and by renal and gastrointestinal excretion.

deposition   **a** Serum calcium is decreased by bone (deposition? resorption?).

excretion   **b** Serum calcium is decreased by gastrointestinal (excretion? resorption?).

excretion   **c** Serum calcium is decreased by renal tubular (resorption? excretion?).

471 The serum calcium level is influenced by both the resorption and the formation of bone. Bone deposition or formation occurs in response to stress and strain.

deposition   Stress and strain on the skeleton results in bone (deposition? resorption?).

472 The major factors that control the serum calcium concentration are vitamin D, parathyroid hormone, calcitonin (thyrocalcitonin), and the serum concentrations of calcium and phosphate ions. Calcitonin (thyrocalcitonin) is a hormone that has a weak effect on extracellular calcium. Calcitonin is secreted by the thyroid gland and reduces the blood calcium concentration.

D   **a** The vitamin that is important in controlling the serum calcium concentration is _____.

parathyroid   **b** The two hormones that are important in the control of serum calcium concentration are _____

calcitonin   and _____.

weak   **c** Calcitonin has a (weak? strong?) effect on the serum calcium concentration.

phosphate   **d** The serum concentrations of calcium and _____ ions influence the serum calcium level.

473 Vitamin D is essential for the regulation of calcium. Vitamin D is ingested in food and is synthesized in the body.

Two sources of vitamin D are

food   **a** _____

synthesis in the body   **b** _____

474 The general actions of vitamin D are to increase calcium absorption from the gastrointestinal tract and to mobilize calcium ions from the bones.

increased

a Absorption of calcium from the gastrointestinal tract is (increased? decreased?) by vitamin D.

calcium

b Vitamin D mobilizes _____ ions from the bones.

475 In addition to vitamin D, parathyroid hormone is important in controlling the serum concentration of calcium. Parathyroid secretion is stimulated by a low serum calcium concentration.

suppress

Because of the feedback mechanism, a high serum calcium concentration would (stimulate? suppress?) parathyroid secretion.

476 One of the functions of parathyroid hormone is to stimulate calcium and phosphate resorption from bone. This would increase the serum calcium concentration.

stimulates

Parathyroid hormone (stimulates? suppresses?) resorption of calcium and phosphate from bone.

477 Parathyroid hormone stimulates resorption of bone, which involves breaking down bone to release calcium and phosphate. Parathyroid hormone also influences the serum calcium concentration through its effect on the kidney to increase the excretion of phosphate ions.

increases

Parathyroid hormone (increases? decreases?) the renal excretion of phosphate ions.

478 Parathyroid hormone reduces the amount of phosphate ions that are resorbed by the kidney tubules. Therefore more phosphate is excreted in the urine and the serum phosphate concentration falls.

less

a Parathyroid hormone influences the kidney tubules to resorb (more? less?) phosphate ions.

falls

b When more phosphate is excreted, the serum phosphate concentration (falls? rises?).

479 Generally speaking, as phosphate levels decrease, serum calcium levels increase.

decrease

Serum calcium levels increase as phosphate levels _____.

480 So far we have considered the effect of vitamin D and of parathyroid hormone on serum calcium levels. Calcitonin inhibits calcium mobilization from bone and therefore tends to lower serum calcium levels in a way that is opposite that of parathyroid hormone. Calcitonin secretion is stimulated directly by a high serum calcium level.

decrease

a The effect of calcitonin is to (increase? decrease?) serum calcium levels.

increase

b The effect of parathyroid hormone is to (increase? decrease?) serum calcium levels.

opposite

c Therefore the effect of calcitonin and of parathyroid hormone on the serum calcium level is (the same? opposite?).

Calcium deficit

481 A serum calcium deficit is called hypocalcemia. In hypocalcemia the serum calcium is below 4.5 mEq/L.

5.3

a Normal serum calcium is 4.5 to _____ mEq/L.

4.5

b In hypocalcemia, the serum calcium is below _____ mEq/L.

482 A serum calcium deficit can occur from inadequate intake or from decreased absorption from the intestine. Persons with pancreatic disease or disease of the small intestine may fail to absorb calcium and will then excrete large amounts of calcium in the feces.

a Serum calcium deficit can occur from inadequate

intake

_____.

b Decreased absorption of calcium from the intestine

hypo-

may result in (hypo-? hyper-?)calcemia.

483 Parathyroid hormone deficiency (hypoparathyroidism) or vitamin D deficiency may result in hypocalcemia. Parathyroid hormone deficiency may develop after thyroid or parathyroid surgery.

a deficit

a Hypocalcemia may be caused by (an excess? a deficit?) of parathyroid hormone.

hypo-

b Vitamin D deficiency may result in (hypo-? hyper-?) calcemia.

484 Rapid dilution of the plasma by intravenous calcium-free solutions may result in hypocalcemia.

hypocalcemia

Giving intravenous fluids rapidly without calcium may result in _____.

485 We have looked at inadequate intake, decreased absorption, pancreatic disease, disease of the small intestine, parathyroid hormone deficiency, vitamin D deficiency, and rapid dilution of the plasma as possible causes of hypocalcemia.

Of the following, which may cause hypocalcemia?

✓   _____ **a** Decreased intestinal absorption

✓   _____ **b** Pancreatic disease

     _____ **c** Hyperactive parathyroids

✓   _____ **d** Vitamin D deficiency

✓   _____ **e** Calcium-free intravenous fluids

486 Other possible causes of hypocalcemia include magnesium deficiency and neoplastic diseases.

deficiency

a Hypocalcemia may be caused by magnesium (deficiency? excess?).

hypo-

b Neoplastic diseases may cause (hypo-? hyper-?)calcemia.

487 Another cause of hypocalcemia is renal insufficiency. When the kidneys are unable to excrete phosphorus normally, hyperphosphatemia results. When the phosphorus rises, the serum calcium level falls.

hypo-

When hyperphosphatemia occurs, (hyper-? hypo-?) calcemia follows.

488 The signs and symptoms of hypocalcemia include those associated with neural excitability. Tetany is the most characteristic sign of hypocalcemia.

tetany

A characteristic sign of hypocalcemia is _____.

489 The signs and symptoms of increased excitability include paresthesias, especially numbness or tingling; skeletal muscle cramps; abdominal spasms and cramps; hyperactive reflexes; and convulsions.

cramps

a Neural excitability that occurs in hypocalcemia may be evidenced by skeletal and abdominal _____.

hyper-

b Reflexes will be (hyper-? hypo-?)active.

490 Trousseau's sign may be present in persons with hypocalcemia. To test for Trousseau's sign, a blood pressure cuff is applied to the upper arm and the cuff is inflated above the systolic level for 3 minutes. A positive sign is the development of carpal spasm (see the illustration below). The person's thumb adducts, and the fingers contract.

a Trousseau's sign may be present in persons with

hypo-
(hypo-? hyper-?)calcemia.

b A positive Trousseau's sign is demonstrated by

carpal spasm
_____.

Carpal spasm. (From Groer, M.W.: Physiology and pathophysiology of the body fluids, St. Louis, 1981, The C.V. Mosby Co.)

491 Chvostek's sign may also be used to observe an increase in neuromuscular excitability. Chvostek's sign is explained in frame 426.

an increase
A positive Chvostek's sign indicates (an increase? a decrease?) in neuromuscular excitability.

492 Mental changes occurring in hypocalcemia may include changes in mood, emotional depression, impairment of memory, confusion, or hallucinations.

hypo-
Emotional depression or confusion may be evidenced in (hypo-? hyper-?)calcemia.

493 If the calcium deficit is prolonged, then calcium will be withdrawn from the bones to increase the extracellular calcium.

In a prolonged calcium deficit, calcium will be mo-
the bones   bilized from _____.

494 It is well established that calcium absorption decreases with aging. The average elderly person in the United States is in negative calcium balance and is losing bone mass. There is growing evidence to indicate that the calcium intake may be inadequate.

decreases   **a** Calcium absorption (increases? decreases?) with aging.

negative   **b** The average elderly person in the United States is in (negative? positive?) calcium balance.

495 By age 70, osteoporosis (loss of density of bone) may result in a decrease in skeletal height. The potential for pathological fractures is increased with osteoporosis. The structural change in skeletal mass may be related to a sedentary life-style, lack of exercise, low calcium intake, vitamin D deficiency, and excessive fat intake.

increased   **a** When osteoporosis is present, the potential for pathological fractures is (increased? decreased?).

may   **b** The loss of skeletal mass (may? may not?) be related to the individuals life-style.

496 The current RDA (recommended dietary allowance) for calcium is 800 mg/day for children and adults and 1200 mg/day for adolescents. There is some evidence to suggest that this should be increased to 1200 to 1500 mg/day for the elderly.

a The current RDA for calcium for children and adults
800   is _____ mg/day.

b The current RDA for calcium for adolescents is
1200   _____ mg/day.

c There is some evidence to suggest that the elderly
1200; 1500   should have a calcium intake of _____ to _____ mg/day.

497 In hypocalcemia a specific abnormal electrocardiographic finding is a prolonged Q-T interval.

An electrocardiographic finding that is characteristic of hypocalcemia is a prolonged _____ interval.

Q-T

498 It is important to observe for hypocalcemia in patients who have had recent surgey involving the thyroid or parathyroid glands. The serum calcium may drop rapidly and result in convulsions.

Following surgery involving the thyroid or parathyroid glands, patients should be observed for signs and symptoms of (hypo-? hyper-?)calcemia.

hypo-

499 Patients who are receiving total parenteral nutrition (hyperalimentation) or who are undergoing hemodialysis should be observed for signs and symptoms of hypocalcemia.

Hypocalcemia may develop in patients who are receiving _____ or who are undergoing _____.

total parenteral nutrition
hemodialysis

500 Acute hypocalcemia is usually treated with a calcium salt, such as calcium gluconate, given intravenously. In cardiac arrest, 10 ml of a 10% solution (4.8 mEq) may be given within a 15- to 30-second period. In situations other than cardiac arrest, 10 ml of a 10% solution should not exceed 0.5 to 1.0 ml/min.

a The calcium salt preferred for treating acute hypocalcemia is _____.

calcium gluconate

b The intravenous rate for 10 ml of a 10% solution of calcium gluconate should not exceed _____ ml/min.

1

501 If the hypocalcemia is mild, a high-calcium diet or oral calcium salts may be given.

Calcium salts (may? may not?) be given orally in mild hypocalcemia.

may

502 In patients who are digitalized, calcium salts should be given cautiously and the patient must be observed continuously on a cardiac monitor. Calcium has an effect on the heart similar to that of digitalis. The arrhythmias that may occur include premature atrial or ventricular contractions, sinus bradycardia, and ventricular tachycardia.

a Calcium has an effect on the heart similar to that of

digitalis

_____.

b A digitalized patient must be observed on a cardiac

calcium

monitor when _____ salts are given intravenously.

503 Whenever calcium salts are being given, you must observe for the signs and symptoms of hypercalcemia. (See frames 513 through 522.)

hypercalcemia

Observe for signs and symptoms of _____ when calcium salts are being given.

SUMMARY

While calcium is the most abundant cation in the body, 99% of the calcium is in the bones. The 1% of calcium in the blood remains remarkably constant. The ionized calcium is needed to help maintain the permeability of cell membranes; for the transmission of nerve impulses and neuromuscular excitability; and for normal cardiac function. Also, calcium is necessary for blood coagulation, activating enzyme reactions, and hormone secretion.

Normally calcium is ingested with the diet and absorbed through the gastrointestinal tract. Serum calcium is gained by resorption of bone and by renal tubular resorption. Serum calcium is lost by renal and gastrointestinal excretion and by bone deposition. Major factors that control the serum calcium concentration are vitamin D, parathyroid hormone, calcitonin, and serum concentrations of calcium and phosphate ions.

A serum calcium deficit can occur from inadequate intake or from decreased absorption. Hypocalcemia may result from a deficiency of parathyroid hormone or of vitamin D. The signs and symptoms of hypocalcemia include those associated with neural excitability. Tetany is the most characteristic sign of hypocalcemia; therefore nursing care must include careful observation to detect increasing neuromuscular excitability. Hypocalcemia is usually treated with a calcium salt, such as calcium gluconate.

REVIEW

calcium

1 The most abundant cation in the body is _____.

essential

2 Calcium is (essential? not essential?) for the transmission of nerve impulses.

3 The most characteristic sign of hypocalcemia is

tetany

_____.

4 In caring for a patient with a potential for hypocalcemia, an important nursing action is _____.

observation

Calcium excess (hypercalcemia)

504 Hypercalcemia exists whenever the serum calcium is over 5.3 mEq/L or 10.6 mg/100 ml.

a Hypocalcemia is indicated by a serum calcium level

4.5

below _____ mEq/L.

5.3

b A serum calcium level over _____ mEq/L indicates hypercalcemia.

505 Hypercalcemia can be the result of excessive intake of calcium, excessive vitamin D intake, or conditions that promote the release of calcium from the bones into the extracellular fluid.

excessive

a Hypercalcemia can result from (excessive? inadequate?) intake of calcium.

hyper-

b Excessive vitamin D intake can result in (hypo-? hyper-?)calcemia.

hypercalcemia

c Conditions that promote the release of calcium from bones can result in _____.

506 Excessive intake of calcium may occur in a person who has peptic ulcer disease and is being treated with milk and alkaline antacids, especially calcium carbonate over a long period of time.

A person with peptic ulcer disease who is treated with milk and calcium carbonate may develop (hyper-?

hyper-

hypo-?)calcemia.

507 Hypercalcemia that develops from vitamin D overdosage occurs primarily because of the increased absorption of calcium from the gastrointestinal tract.

Excessive vitamin D may result in hypercalcemia because of (increased? decreased?) absorption of calcium from the intestine.

increased

508 Several conditions may cause increased release of calcium from bones and thus result in hypercalcemia. The most common cause of hypercalcemia is cancer. Hypercalcemia can be a complication of almost any malignant disorder, but it is especially frequent in cancer of the breast. Bone metastasis may result in breakdown of normal bone and release of excessive calcium.

a Increased release of calcium from bone may cause (hypo? hyper-?)calcemia.

hyper-

b The most common cause of hypercalcemia is

cancer

_____.

c Hypercalcemia is especially frequent in cancer of the

breast

_____.

509 While metastasis to bone may cause breakdown of bone and release of excessive calcium, cancer may cause hypercalcemia without bone metastasis. Many malignant tumors produce inappropriate hormones. Certain tumors produce a parathyroid-like substance, which causes increased bone resorption and a rise in the serum calcium concentration.

Causes of release of excessive calcium from bone include

metastasis

a cancer with _____ to bone

parathyroid

b production of a _____ -like hormone from the tumor

510 Bone destruction may exceed bone production to the extent that the kidneys are unable to excrete the excessive calcium ions. Also, hypercalcemia may result from a primary hyperparathyroidism, which may be caused by a benign adenoma of one or more parathyroid glands.

a Primary hyperparathyroidism may be caused by a

benign

_____ adenoma.

b Hyperparathyroidism will result in (hypo-? hyper-?) calcemia.

511 Another cause of hypercalcemia is prolonged immobilization. Remember, we learned that bone deposition or formation occurs in response to stress and strain (frame 471). Therefore with disuse there is increased bone resorption, but bone formation is also decreased.

a Prolonged immobilization may result in (hyper-? hypo-?)calcemia.

b Disuse causes (increased? decreased?) bone resorption.

c Disuse results in (increased? decreased?) bone formation.

512 In considering the causes of hypercalcemia, we have looked at factors related to excessive intake of calcium, increased bone destruction, and decreased bone formation. There are other causes of hypercalcemia, such as the use of diuretics, endocrine disorders, and renal diseases.

Factors that lead to hypercalcemia include the following:

_____ **a** Excessive intake of calcium

_____ **b** Decreased bone destruction

_____ **c** Decreased bone formation

_____ **d** Use of diuretics

_____ **e** Renal diseases

513 The signs and symptoms of hypercalcemia result from three sources: a decrease in neuromuscular activity, resorption of calcium from bone, and the effect on the kidney of high calcium concentrations.

Three sources for the signs and symptoms of hypercalcemia include

a (a decrease? an increase?) in neuromuscular activity

b (resorption? deposition?) of calcium from/in bone

c effect on the kidney of (high? low?) calcium concentration

514 The decreased neuromuscular activity will be evidenced in generalized muscle weakness, lethargy, loss of muscle tone, and ataxia. The person may show mental confusion, impairment of memory, slurred speech, personality or behavior changes, stupor, or coma.

decreased

hyper-

a In hypercalcemia generalized muscle weakness results from the (increased? decreased?) neuromuscular activity.

b Stupor or coma may result from (hypo-? hyper-?)calcemia.

515 The heart responds to hypercalcemia with effects that look like digitalis effect. Bradycardia and increased contractility occur in hypercalcemia. In the electrocardiogram, the Q-T interval shortens and the T waves invert. Ventricular arrhythmias may develop.

brady-

shortens

arrhythmias

a Cardiac effects of hypercalcemia may include (brady-? tachy-?)cardia.

b The Q-T interval on the electrocardiogram (lengthens? shortens?).

c With hypercalcemia, ventricular _____ may develop.

516 The gastrointestinal symptoms of hypercalcemia include anorexia, nausea, vomiting, and constipation.

constipation

Hypercalcemia may have symptoms including anorexia, nausea, vomiting, and (constipation? diarrhea?).

517 The signs and symptoms related to resorption of calcium from bone include deep bone pain and radiographic evidence of bone demineralization.

calcium

Deep bone pain may be caused by resorption of _____ from the bone.

518 High extracellular concentrations of calcium impair the ability of the kidney to concentrate urine.

polyuria

When the kidney is less able to concentrate urine, (polyuria? anuria?) will be evident.

519 The polyuria that results from hypercalcemia will lead to the need for increased intake of water.

will

Polyuria (will? will not?) lead to the need for increased water intake.

520 Hypercalcemia will predispose to the development of renal calculi (kidney stones).

Renal calculi may be the result of (hyper-? hypo-?) calcemia.

521 Hypercalcemic crisis is an emergency condition caused by an acute increase in serum calcium levels above 8 to 9 mEq/L (17 mg/100 ml). Hypercalcemic crisis has signs and symptoms of intractable nausea, dehydration, stupor, and coma. Azotemia is present. Hypokalemia and/or hypomagnesemia may be present along with hypernatremia because of the water loss.

a Hypercalcemic crisis may occur if the serum calcium rises above _____ to _____ mEq/L.

8; 9

b The intractable nausea and vomiting will lead to a (deficit? excess?) in fluid volume.

deficit

c Another electrolyte imbalance likely to be present is (hypo-? hyper-?)kalemia.

hypo-

522 With hypercalcemic crisis, mortality has been high. Death often results from cardiac arrest.

Mortality is (high? low?) in hypercalcemic crisis.

high

523 Treating hypercalcemia involves removing the cause or controlling the condition that caused the excess serum calcium. When hypercalcemia is severe, the first thing to receive attention is the need for hydration. This will reduce the risk of renal damage and may reduce the serum calcium by dilution.

When hypercalcemia is severe, _____ must be adequate to reduce the possible renal damage.

hydration

524 Normal saline given intravenously will provide hydration as well as produce some urinary excretion of calcium, since the kidneys selectively resorb sodium.

The intravenous solution used to provide hydration in hypercalcemia is _____.

normal saline

525 When normal saline is given intravenously, it is important to match the rate and amount of saline solution to the patient's urine output. You need to measure the patient's hourly, as well as total, urine output.

When normal saline is given intravenously to treat hypercalcemia, you should measure the urine output _____ (frequency).

hourly

526 If normal saline does not produce adequate diuresis, then diuretics such as furosemide (Lasix) may be given to increase the excretion of calcium.

Diuretics such as _____ may be used to increase the excretion of calcium.

furosemide (Lasix)

527 Phosphate may be used to lower the serum calcium level. Phosphate acts by promoting deposition of calcium in bone and decreasing intestinal absorption. A side effect of oral phosphate ingestion is diarrhea. Intravenous infusions of phosphate are used only for hypercalcemic crisis because of the potential for soft tissue calcification and potential renal failure if the serum calcium decreases acutely.

a The substance that acts by promoting deposition of calcium in bone and decreases intestinal absorption is _____.

phosphate

b Intravenous infusions of phosphate are used only for _____ crisis.

hypercalcemic

528 Corticosteroids (Cortef) and mithramycin (Mithracin) are used for treating hypercalcemia in persons with cancer. Mithramycin is a potent antitumor drug that shares the cytotoxicities of other antitumor drugs but does lower serum calcium concentration.

Corticosteroids and mithramycin are used for treating hypercalcemia in persons with _____.

cancer

529 In giving care to a person with hypercalcemia, it is important to protect him from pathological fractures. Positioning and moving must be done with extreme care to prevent fractures.

A potental problem for persons with hypercalcemia is pathological _____.

fractures

530 Formation of calcium stones in the urinary tract is another potential problem for persons with hypercalcemia. Persons with hypercalcemia should be encouraged to drink 3000 to 4000 ml of water per day to reduce the possibility of renal calculi.

a Persons with hypercalcemia may develop _____ in the urinary tract.

calculi

3000
4000

b Persons with hypercalcemia should drink _____ to _____ ml of water per day.

531 Acidic urine will help to decrease the possibility of urinary stone formation. Foods such as prunes or cranberry juice or ascorbic acid will favor increased acidity in the urine.

alkaline

a Urinary stone formation is more likely in (acidic? alkaline?) urine.

b Persons with hypercalcemia should eat foods that will

acidic

help produce (acidic? alkaline?) urine.

532 Urinary tract infections should be avoided. Good perineal care and meticulous catheter care are especially important for persons with hypercalcemia.

Good perineal care and meticulous catheter care will

infections

help prevent urinary tract _____.

SUMMARY

Hypercalcemia can be the result of excessive calcium intake, excessive vitamn D intake, or conditons that promote release of calcium from the bones. Whenever bone destruction exceeds bone production to the extent that the kidneys are unable to excrete the excess calcium ions, hypercalcemia may result.

The signs and symptoms of hypercalcemia result from a decrease in neuromuscular activity, resorption of calcium from bone, and the effect on the kidney of high serum calcium concentrations. The decreased neuromuscular activity may be evidenced by generalized muscle weakness, loss of muscle tone, mental confusion, and coma. The cardiac signs of hypercalcemia include bradycardia, increased contractility, and ventricular arrhythmias. The increased resorption of bone is evidenced by deep bone pain and radiographic evidence of bone demineralization. The effect on the kidney is indicated by decreased concentration of urine, increased urine output, and renal calculi.

Hypercalcemic crisis is caused by a rapid increase in

serum calcium levels to above 8 to 9 mEq/L. Adequate hydration must be provided. Diuretics and/or phosphate may be used to treat hypercalcemic crisis.

In caring for patients with hypercalcemia, it is important to protect them from pathological fractures. Urinary tract infections should be prevented. Intake of water should be in amounts of 3000 to 4000 ml/day.

REVIEW

1 Three causes of hypercalcemia include

excessive intake   **a** _____

excessive vitamin D   **b** _____

release of calcium from bone   **c** _____

a decrease

2 The signs and symptoms of hypercalcemia include (a decrease? an increase?) in neuromuscular activity.

3 The increased resorption of bone is evidenced by

deep bone pain   **a** _____

radiographic evidence of de-mineralization   **b** _____

pathological fractures

4 Patients with hypercalcemia should be moved gently because of the potential for _____.

3000; 4000

5 A patient with hypercalcemia should have a daily fluid intake of _____ to _____ ml.

Bibliography

1. Anthony, C.P., and Thibodeau, G.A.: Textbook of anatomy and physiology, ed.11, St. Louis, 1983, The C.V. Mosby Co.
2. Behrman, R.E., and Vaughn, V.C.: Nelson textbook of pediatrics, ed. 12, Philadelphia, 1983, W.B. Saunders Co.
3. Beland, I.L.: Clinical nursing, ed. 4, New York, 1981, MacMillan Publishing Co.
4. Brocklehurst, J.C.: Textbook of geriatric medicine and gerontology, New York, 1985, Churchill Livingstone.
5. Brunner, L.S., Emerson, P.E., Jr., Ferguson, L.K., and Suddarth, D.S.: Textbook of medical-surgical nursing, ed. 5, Philadelphia, 1984, J.B. Lippincott Co.
6. Burke, S.R.: The composition and function of body fluids, ed. 3, St. Louis, 1980, The C.V. Mosby Co.
7. Ganong, W.F.: Review of medical physiology, ed. 12, Los Altos, Calif., 1985, Lange Medical Publications.
8. Goldberger, E.A.: A primer of water, electrolyte and acid-base syndromes, ed. 7, Philadelphia, 1986, Lea & Febiger.
9. Goodhart, R.S., and Shils, M.E.: Modern nutrition in health and disease, ed 6, Philadelphia, 1980, Lea & Febiger.
10. Groer, M.W.: Physiology and pathophysiology of the body fluids, St. Louis, 1981, The C.V. Mosby Co.
11. Guyton, A.C.: Textbook of medical physiology, ed. 6, Philadelphia, 1981, W.B. Saunders Co.
12. Hazinski, M.F.: Nursing care of the critically ill child, St. Louis, 1984, The C.V. Mosby Co.
13. Lentner, C., editor: Geigy scientific tables, vol. 1, units of measurement; body fluids; composition of the body; nutrition, ed. 8, Summit, N.J., 1981, Ciba-Geigy Corp.
14. Kaplan, L.C., and Pesce, A.J.: Clinical chemistry: theory, analysis and correlation, St. Louis, 1984, The C.V. Mosby Co.
15. Luckman, J., and Sorenson, K.C.: Medical-surgical nursing, ed. 2, Philadelphia, 1980, W.B. Saunders Co.
16. Lye, M.: Electrolyte disorders in the elderly, Clin. Endocrinol. Metab. 13(2):377, 1984.
17. Martof, M.: Fluid balance, part 1, J. Nephrol. Nurs. 2(1):10, 1985.
18. Maxwell, M.H., and Kleeman, C.R.: Clinical disorders of fluid and electrolyte metabolism, ed. 4, New York, 1986, McGraw-Hill Book Co.
19. Meites, S.: Pediatric clinicial chemistry, Washington, D.C., 1981, The American Association for Clinical Chemistry.
20. Mountcastle, V.B.: Medical physiology, ed. 14, St. Louis, 1980, The C.V. Mosby Co.
21. Murray, R.B., Huelskoetter, M.M.W., and O'Driscol, D.L.: The nursing process in later maturity, New Jersey, 1980, Prentice-Hall, Inc.
22. Olds, S.B., London, M., Ladewig, P.A., and Davidson, S.V.: Maternal-Newborn nursing, San Fransisco, 1980, Addison-Wesley Publishing Co.
23. Perry, A.G., and Potter, P.A.: Clinical nursing skills and techniques, St. Louis, 1986, The C.V. Mosby Co.

24. Phillips, P.A., et. al.: Reduced thirst after water deprivation in healthy elderly men, N. Engl. J. Med. **311**(2):753, 1984.
25. Phipps, W.J., Long, B.C., and Woods, N.F.: Medical-surgical nursing: concepts and clinical practice, ed. 3, St. Louis, 1987, The C.V. Mosby Co.
26. Plumer, A.L.: Principles and practice of intravenous therapy, ed. 3, Boston, 1982, Little, Brown & Co.
27. Porth, C.: Pathophysiology: concepts of altered health states, Philadelphia, 1982, J.B. Lippincott Co.
28. Ramsey, J.M.: Basic pathophysiology, Palo Alto, Calif., 1982, Addison-Wesley Publishing Co.
29. Rose, B.D.: Clinical physiology of acid-base and electrolyte disorders, ed. 2, New York, 1984, McGraw-Hill Book Co.
30. Shapiro, B.A., Harrison, R.A., and Walton, J.R.: Clinical application of blood gases, ed. 3, Chicago, 1982, Year Book Medical Publishers, Inc.
31. Sodeman, W.A., Jr., and Sodeman, W.A.: Pathologic physiology: mechanisms of disease, ed. 6, Philadelphia, 1979, W.B. Saunders Co.
32. Tilkian, S.M., Conover, M.B., and Tilkian, A.G.: Clinical implications of laboratory tests, ed. 4, St. Louis, 1987, The C.V. Mosby Co.
33. Underhill, S.L., Woods, S., Sivarajan, E.S., and Halpenny, C.J.: Cardiac nursing, Philadelphia, 1982, J.B. Lippincott Co.
34. Whaley, L.F., and Wong, D.L.: Nursing care of infants and children, ed. 3, St. Louis, 1987, The C.V. Mosby Co.
35. Widmann, F.W.: Clinical interpretation of laboratory tests, ed. 9, Philadelphia, 1983, F.A. Davis Co.
36. Wyngaarden, J.B., and Smith, L.H.: Cecil textbook of medicine, ed. 17, Philadelphia, 1985, W.B. Saunders Co.

Index

A

Abbott administration set, 98
Abdomen, fluid in, 110–111
  and hypernatremia, 125
Abdominal distention and hypokalemia, 135
Abdominal pain from metabolic acidosis, 71
Abdominal spasms and cramps and hypo-
      calcemia, 167
Abdominal surgery and fluid volume shift,
      110–111
Acetic acid, 44
Acetoacetic acid and metabolic acidosis, 60
Acid, 44–45
  acetic, 44
  acetoacetic, and metabolic acidosis, 60
  carbonic; *see* Carbonic acid
  hydrochloric, 44, 50
    as buffer, 50
    loss of, causing metabolic alkalosis, 73
  hydrogen ions and, 44
  strong, 44
  sulfuric, 44
  weak, 44
Acid-base balance, 43
  age and, 53–54
  electrolytes and, 115
Acid-base buffer, 49
Acid-base imbalance, 43–81
  clinical conditions of, 56–65
  combination of types of, 64
  nursing care in, 66–77
  nursing responsibilities in, 73–75
Acidic solution, 45

Acidic urine, 53
Acidity, 44
  determination of, 44
  and pH value, 44
Acidosis, 48, 56
  central nervous system effects of, 46, 64
  death from, 46
  diabetic, 61, 62
  effect of
    on body, 64
    on nervous system, 65
  metabolic; *see* Metabolic acidosis
  pH level in, 66
  renal tubular, and hypokalemia, 133–134
  respiratory; *see* Respiratory acidosis
  respiratory system and, 51–52
  uremic, causing metabolic acidosis, 60
Active transport system, 21
Addison's disease and potassium level, 140
Adenoma, parathyroid, and hypercalcemia,
    173
ADH; *see* Antidiuretic hormone
Administration of fluids
  adjusting, 101–103
  calculating, 98–99
  mechanical factors affecting, 100
  nurse's responsibilities in, 95–97
  rate of flow in, 96–97
Adrenal cortical insufficiency
  and fluid volume excess, 105
  and hyperkalemia, 140
Adrenal cortical steroid hormones and po-
    tassium excretion, 134

Adrenal corticoids and hypernatremia, 124
Adrenal glands
  overactive, 38
  and sodium balance, 116
  underactive, 38
Adults
  distribution of body fluids in, 1, 4–5
  fluid requirements for, 91–92
Age and acid-base balance, 53–54
Agitation and hypomagnesemia, 152
Airway, foreign objects in, causing respiratory acidosis, 68
Albumin, calcium and, 162
Alcoholism and hypomagnesemia, 149
Aldactone; see Spironolactone
Aldosterone
  effect of, on sodium absorption, 117, 127
  and fluid volume regulation, 36, 37–38
  and hypokalemia, 134
  overproduction of
    and hypernatremia, 124, 127
    treatment of, 127
  potassium regulation by, 131–132
  secretion of
    and fluid volume, 83
    rate of, 117
  and sodium balance regulation, 116–117
Aldosteronism, primary, and hypomagnesemia, 150
Alkaline solution, 44, 45
Alkaline urine, 53, 59
Alkalinity, 44
  determination of, 44
  and pH level, 44
Alkalosis, 48
  body potassium level and, 131
  central nervous system effects of, 46–64
  effect of, on body, 64
  and hypokalemia, 132
  metabolic; see Metabolic alkalosis
  peripheral nervous system excitation and, 64
  pH level of, 66
  respiratory; see Respiratory alkalosis
  serum potassium and, 132
Altitude, high, respiratory alkalosis from, 58
Amines, pressor, for hyponatremia, 121–122
Analgesics and antidiuretic hormone secretion, 104–105

Anesthetics and antidiuretic hormone secretion, 104
Angiotensin, formation of, 117
Anion(s), 7–8, 9
  attraction of, to anode, 8, 9
  availability of, 10
  charge of, 7–8
  electrical attraction of, 8, 9
  electrode attraction of, 8
Anode, 8
Anorexia
  and hypercalcemia, 175
  and hypokalemia, 135
  and hyponatremia, 119
Anoxia and oxygen usage, 70
Antidiuretic hormone
  decreased secretion of, and fluid volume excess, 104
  excessive secretion of
    causes of, 104–105
    and fluid volume excess, 104
  and fluid volume regulation, 36, 37, 38–39
  lack of, 85
  and regulation of fluid balance, 83
  and urine volume regulation, 83
Anxiety and respiratory acidosis, 68
Apathy and sodium loss, 119
Aphasia as sign of fluid volume excess, 106
Apnea and hypokalemia, 135
Aramine; see Metaraminol
Arrest
  cardiac, from potassium administration, 137
  respiratory, from hypokalemia, 135
  systolic, and hypokalemia, 135–136
Arrhythmias
  from calcium and digitalis, 170–171
  from respiratory acidosis, 68
  from respiratory alkalosis, 70
  ventricular, and hypercalcemia, 175
Arterial blood gas analysis, 66
Arterial carbon dioxide tension, 66; see also PCO_2
Arterial oxygen tension, 66
Arterial pressure
  and extracellular fluid volume, 36
  and sodium balance, 116
Arteriosclerosis, cerebral, and water deficit, 85

Ascites, 110
and hypernatremia, 125
Aspirin overdose, respiratory alkalosis from, 58–59
Ataxia and hypercalcemia, 174
Athetoid movements and hypomagnesemia, 157
Atom, 6
charge of, 6–7
electrical charge of, 6–7; *see also* Ion(s)
neutral, 7
nucleus of, 5
particles of, 6
Atrial contractions, premature
from calcium and digitalis, 170–171
and hypomagnesemia, 152
Atropine and thirst, 36
Attention, loss of, and fluid volume excess, 106
Azotemia in hypercalcemic crisis, 176

B

B vitamins and magnesium, 146
Babinski's sign, positive, and hypomagnesemia, 151
Bag inhalation of carbon dioxide for respiratory alkalosis, 71
Balance
acid-base; *see* Acid-base balance
fluid and electrolyte, 1–42
controls for maintaining, 34–39
Base, 44–45
hydrogen ions and, 44
Base bicarbonate, 49
symbol for, 62
Baxter administration set, 98
Behavior, unusual, and fluid volume excess, 106
Bicarbonate
for respiratory acidosis, 58
serum level of, in hyponatremia, 121
standard plasma, measurement of, 66–67
Bicarbonate ions and hydrogen ion balance, 53
Bicarbonate-carbonic acid system, 49, 50–51
Bicarbonate-carbonic acid buffer system; *see also* Carbonate buffer system
Blood
coagulation of, calcium and, 163

Blood—cont'd
hydrostatic pressure of, 24
osmotic pressure of, 24
Blood flow through kidneys, decreased, and fluid volume excess, 104
Blood gas analysis, 66–67
arterial, 66
summary of, 68
Blood pressure
in hypovolemia, 111–112
during magnesium infusion, 155
Blood volume and extracellular fluid volume, 36
Body, water and electrolytes entering and leaving, normal mechanisms for, 28–32
Body fluid(s); *see also* Fluid(s); Water
balance of, with electrolytes, controls for maintaining, 34–39
composition of, imbalance in, 33
concentration of, imbalance in, 32–33
concentration of constituents in, 2
constituents of, 6–12
deficit of, 1
causes of, 82
laboratory findings in, 83–84
patients likely to have, 85, 91
signs and symptoms of, 84–90, 91
in infant, 91
distribution of
in adults, 1, 4
electrolytes and, 115
electrolytes in; *see* Electrolyte(s)
excess of
hematocrit level in, 107
hemoglobin level in, 107
signs and symptoms of, 106–108
treatment of, 108
and weight gain, 106
excretion of, 5
extracellular; *see* Extracellular body fluid
functions of, 2
homeostasis of; *see* Homeostasis
illness and, 81
ingestion of liquids as source of, 5
interstitial; *see* Interstitial body fluid
intracellular; *see* Intracellular body fluid
intravascular; *see* Intravascular body fluid

Body fluid(s)—cont'd
  metabolism as source of, 5
  movement of, 14–28
    control of, in and out of cells, 129
  nutrient transportation in, 2
  percentage of body weight in, 1, 4–5
  replacing, 1
  replenishment of, 5
  resorption of, 112
  retention of; *see* Edema
  sources of, 82
  specific gravity of, 20–21
  units of measurement of, 9–11
  volume of
    deficit in, 82–104
    excess of, 104–110
      causes of, 104
      signs and symptoms of, 106–108
      treatment of, 108
    imbalance in, 32, 81–114
    measurement of, 9
    shifts in, 110–113
    sodium and, 116, 117
    tests indicating, 84
  waste product transportation in, 2
Body fluid compartments, 2–4
  electrolyte composition of, 12–14
  semipermeable membranes separating, 3
Body weight, fluid percentage of, 1, 4–5
Bone(s)
  calcium in, 162–163
  demineralization of, and hypercalcemia,
      175
  deposition of, and calcium, 164
  destruction of, and hypercalcemia, 174
  formation of, and hypercalcemia, 174
Bone pain, deep, and hypercalcemia, 175
Bottle of intravenous fluids
  height of, and flow rate, 100
  labeling of, 101
Bowel obstruction and hyponatremia, 118
Bowel resection and hypomagnesemia, 149
Bradycardia
  and hypercalcemia, 175
  sinus, from calcium and digitalis, 170–
      171
Breast cancer causing hypercalcemia, 173
Breath, shortness of
  and intravenous infusion, 102
  as symptom of congestive heart failure, 96

Breathing; *see also* Respiratory system
  hyperactive, 61, 62
  Kussmaul, 61, 62
  shallow and slow, from metabolic alka-
      losis, 63
Buffer, 49
  acid-base, 49
Buffer system, 48, 49–51, 56
  carbonate; *see* Carbonate buffer system
  summary of, 54
Burns
  body fluid loss due to, 1, 85, 92
  and hyponatremia, 118

C

Calcitonin and serum calcium, 164, 166
Calcium
  absorption of, 163–165
  and albumin, 162
  in body, 161
  bound to protein, 161–162
  deficit of, 166–172; *see also* Hypocal-
      cemia
  digitalis and, 170–171
  excess of, 172–179; *see also* Hypercal-
      cemia
  excessive intake of, 172
    and hypomagnesemia, 149
  functions of, 162–163
  imbalance of, 161–179
  ionized, 161–162
  loss of, 164
  and magnesium, 146
  mobilization of, from bone, 169, 173
  normal level of, 166
  and phosphate, 164, 165
  RDA for, 169
  release of excessive levels of, from bone,
      173
  serum concentration of, factors control-
      ling, 164–165
Calcium bicarbonate, 49
Calcium carbonate for peptic ulcer disease,
    172
Calcium gluconate
  for hyperglycemia, 143
  for hypermagnesemia, 160, 161
  for hypocalcemia, 170
Calcium salts for hypocalcemia, 170
Calculi, renal, and hypercalcemia, 175–176

Cancer
  breast, causing hypercalcemia, 173
  causing hypercalcemia, 173
  lung, and antidiuretic hormone secretion,
    105
Capillaries
  increased permeability of, and "third spac-
    ing," 111
  liver, 25
  venous end of
    hydrostatic pressure at, 24–25
    osmotic pressure at, 24–25
Capillary walls, permeability of, 14, 25
  and "third spacing," 111
Carbohydrates
  for diabetic acidosis, 61
  metabolism of, and magnesium, 146, 147
Carbon dioxide
  bag inhalation of, for respiratory alkalosis,
    71
  and carbonic acid formation, 52
  content of, measurement of, 66–67
  5%, for respiratory alkalosis, 71
  formation of, in body, 51
  loss of, in respiratory alkalosis, 58
  partial pressure of; see PCO_2
Carbon dioxide tension, arterial, 66
Carbonate buffer system, 49–50, 56
Carbonic acid, 44, 49, 50
  concentration of, in respiratory acidosis,
    68–69
  formation of, 52
  and respiratory acidosis, 57–58
  symbol for, 62
Carbonic acid-sodium bicarbonate buffer
    system, 49–50, 56
Cardiac arrest from potassium administra-
    tion, 137
Cardiac function and calcium, 163
Cardiac standstill from hyperkalemia, 141
Cardiovascular signs of hyponatremia, 120
Carpal spasm and hypocalcemia, 168
Cathartics, magnesium-containing, and hy-
    permagnesemia, 158–159
Catheterization of patient in acid-base im-
    balance, 75
Cathode, 8, 9
Cations, 7, 8, 9
  attraction of, to cathode, 8, 9
  availability of, 10

Cations—cont'd
  charge of, 7
  movement of, control of, 129
Cation-exchange resins for hyperkalemia,
    143
Cell(s)
  chemical composition of, 2
  concentration of constituents of, 2
  crenated, 19, 82
  hypotonic solution causing swelling of, 19
  shrinkage of, 19, 104
  size of, and sodium, 116, 129
  swelling of, from fluid volume excess, 104
Cell membranes
  nerve excitability of, calcium and, 162
  permeability of, calcium and, 163
  permeable, 15, 16
  selectively permeable, 15, 16
  semipermeable, 15, 16
Cellular crenation, 82
Cellular dehydration, 82
Central nervous system
  in acidosis, 64
  depression of, 64
  and pH, 46
Central venous pressure in hypovolemia,
    112
Cerebral arteriosclerosis and water deficit,
    85
Cerebral function, disturbed, symptoms of,
    110
Cerebral injury and water deficit, 85
Cerebral lesions and antidiuretic hormone se-
    cretion, 105
Chemical activity of electrolytes, 9–10
Child(ren)
  fluid requirements for, 92–94
  and fluid volume excess, 104
  hematocrit in, 84
  infusion rates for, 97
  loss of skin turgor in, with sodium deficit,
    119–120
  maintenance fluids in, calculation of, 29
  potassium infusion in, 137
  potassium levels in, 129
Chloride
  as anion, 8
  charge of, 8
  loss of, 62–63
  and resorption of sodium, 116–117

Chloride—cont'd
  serum level of, in hyponatremia, 121
Chloride-containing solutions for metabolic alkalosis, 73
Choreiform movements and hypomagnesemia, 151
Chvostek's sign
  and hypocalcemia, 168
  and hypomagnesemia, 151
Circulatory failure and hypokalemia, 136
Cirrhosis of liver; see Liver cirrhosis
Clonus and hypomagnesemia, 151
Coagulation, blood, calcium and, 163
Colloid osmotic pressure, 23
  and hydrostatic pressure, 24
Coma
  from acidosis, 46, 64
  and fluid volume deficit, 85
  from fluid volume excess, 106, 108
  and hypercalcemia, 175
  in hypercalcemic crisis, 176
  from hypermagnesemia, 159, 160
Combining power of electrolytes, 9–10
Compartments, body fluid; see Body fluid compartments
Compensated metabolic acidosis, 72
Confusion
  in hypercalcemia, 174–175
  in hypocalcemia, 168
  from hypomagnesemia, 152, 156
  from metabolic acidosis, 71
  from metabolic alkalosis, 73
  and potassium depletion, 135
  and respiratory acidosis, 68
  as sign of body water deficit, 86
  as sign of fluid volume excess, 106
Congestive heart failure, 25–26
  and fluid volume excess, 105
  and hypernatremia, 124
  from ingestion of fluid, 95–96
  symptoms of, 96
Consciousness, assessment of, in acid-base imbalance, 74
Constipation and hypercalcemia, 175
Contractility of heart, increased, and hypercalcemia, 175
Contractions, premature atrial or ventricular
  from calcium and digitalis, 170–171
  and hypomagnesemia, 152

Convulsions
  from acid-base imbalance, 75
  and alkalosis, 46, 64
  and fluid volume excess, 106, 107, 108
  and hypocalcemia, 167, 170
  and hypomagnesemia, 151, 156
  in toxemia of pregnancy, magnesium and, 146
Cortef; see Corticosteroids
Corticosteroids for hypercalcemia, 177
Cortisone and hypokalemia, 134
Coughing
  as symptom of congestive heart failure, 96
  as symptom of pulmonary edema, 102
Cramps
  and hypocalcemia, 167
  and hypokalamia, 135
  and hyponatremia, 119
Creatinine in solution, 6
Crenated cells, 19
Crenation, cellular, 82
Crush injuries and hyperkalemia, 140
Cubic centimeter, 9
Cushing's syndrome, 38
Cutter administration set, 98
Cyanosis
  as symptom of congestive heart failure, 96
  as symptom of pulmonary edema, 90
Cystic fibrosis and hyponatremia, 118

D
Death
  from fluid volume excess, 106
  from hypercalcemia crisis, 176
  from hypokalemia, 135
  from pH imbalance, 45
Deep tendon reflexes, loss of, from hypermagnesemia, 159, 160
Defense mechanisms of body, 48–56
Dehydration, 86–87
  cellular, 82
  in hypercalcemic crisis, 176
  and hypermagnesemia, 159
  hypernatremia causing symptoms of, 125
  hypertonic, 87
    physical signs of, 88
  hypotonic, 87
    physical signs of, 88
  isotonic, 87, 88
    physical signs of, 88

Delirium as sign of body water deficit, 86
Demerol; *see* Meperidine
Demineralization, bone, and hypercalcemia, 175
Depression
  in hypocalcemia, 168
  and hypomagnesemia, 152
  respiratory, from hypermagnesemia, 159, 160
Diabetes insipidus and water loss, 85
Diabetes mellitus causing metabolic acidosis, 60
Diabetic acidosis, 61, 62
Diabetic ketoacidosis and hypermagnesemia, 150, 159
Dialysis
  for hypermagnsemia, 160
  peritoneal, for hyperkalemia, 143
Diaphoresis
  from hypermagnesemia, 159
  during magnesium infusion, 155, 156
Diaphragm, paralysis of, and hypokalemia, 135
Diarrhea
  and body fluid loss, 30, 92
  causing metabolic acidosis, 60
  effect of, on fluid balance, 20
  and hypokalemia, 133, 134, 139
  and hypomagnesemia, 149
  and hyponatremia, 118
  from magnesium salts, 153
  from phosphate ingestion, 177
Diffusion, 14–16, 26, 27
  molecule and ion movement in, 21–22
  of water through skin, 29
Digitalis
  and calcium, 110–111
  and hypokalemia, 136
  and hypomagnesemia, 150, 153
Disease
  and fluid volume shift, 111
  kidney; *see* Kidney, disease of
  lung, chronic obstructive, 79
  neoplastic
    and hypocalcemia, 167
    with metastasis to bone, 153
  pancreatic, and hypocalcemia, 166, 167
  peptic ulcer, and hypercalcemia, 172
  of small intestine, and hypocalcemia, 166, 167

Disorientation and respiratory acidosis, 68
Dissociation of electrolytes, 8
Distilled water, 18–19
  oral intake of, 94
Distressed respiration and respiratory acidosis, 68
Diuretics
  and hypercalcemia, 174, 177
  for hypernatremia, 126
  and hypokalemia, 134
  and hypomagnesemia, 150
  nursing responsibility with, 126
  potassium-sparing, 134
Drinking water, 94
  to correct fluid volume deficit, 83
Drop factor, 99
Drop size in intravenous administration set, 98–99
Drowsiness from hypermagnesemia, 159

E

Edema, 37, 42
  in abdominal cavity, 125
  and fluid volume excess, 107
  and hypernatremia, 124
  and hyponatremia, 118
  pulmonary; *see* Pulmonary edema
  and sodium excess, 124, 125
Elderly
  calcium deficit in, 169
  dehydration in, 89–90
  fluid balance in, 1
  fluid requirements for, 94
  and fluid volume deficit, 84
  and fluid volume excess, 104
  and fluid volume imbalance, 81–82
  hypernatremia in, 124
  hypokalemia in, 134
  intracellular fluid of, 5
  and sodium imbalance, 117
  thirst sensation in, 83
Electrocardiogram
  effects of hypercalcemia on, 175
  effects of hyperkalemia on, 135–136, 141–142
Electrolyte(s), 6–12
  action of, 9–10
  active transport system of, 21
  availability of, 10
  balance of, with fluids, 1–42

Electrolyte(s)—cont'd
  balance of, with fluids—cont'd
    controls for maintaining, 34–39
  chemical activity of, 10
  combining power of, 9–10
  composition of, in body fluid compartments, 12–14
  concentration deficit of, 40
  dissociation of, 8
  entering body, 28
  excretion of, 28–29
  and fluid imbalance, 39–42
  functions of, in body, 115
  imbalance in, 115–179
  loss of, 82
  measurement of, 9–11
  and water entering and leaving body, normal mechanisms for, 28–32
Electron, 6
  charge of, 6–7
  position of, in atom, 6–7
Emphysema
  carbon dioxide level in, 56–58
  causing respiratory acidosis, 68
Encephalitis, respiratory alkalosis from, 58
Endocrine disorders and hypercalcemia, 174
Energy, loss of, and hyponatremia, 121
Enzyme reactions, activation of
  calcium and, 163
  magnesium and, 146, 147
Equilibrium, osmotic, 18
Equivalent, weight, 10
Excitability of nerve tissue
  and calcium, 163
  and hypocalcemia, 167
Extracellular body fluid, 2, 3
  composition of
    changes in, and sodium balance, 116
    imbalance in, 41–42
  concentration of sodium in, 21
  concentration imbalance of, 40
  excess; see Body fluid(s), excess of
  extraction of water from, 82
  hypertonic, 82
  mixing, 3
  osmolality of, 20–21
  osmotic balance of, with intracellular fluid, 84–85
  pH of, determination of, 48

Extracellular body fluid—cont'd
  volume of
    decrease in, stimulating thirst, 35–36
    deficit of, 40
    imbalance of, 39–40
    increased, 124
    influence of sodium excess on, 124
    and kidneys, 36
    sodium and, 116
Extracellular compartments, 3–4
Eyeballs, changes in, in sodium deficit, 120

F

Fainting and hyponatremia, 121
Fatigue
  and hypokalemia, 135
  and hyponatremia, 119, 120
Fear and antidiuretic hormone secretion, 104
Feces, loss of water through, 30
Fever
  causing respiratory alkalosis, 58, 70
  and fluid requirements, 92
  and hypernatremia, 125
  and water loss, 85
Fibrillation, ventricular, from respiratory acidosis, 68
Filtration, 22–23, 27, 28
Filtration force, 24
  net, 24
Fingers; see Tingling sensations
Fistula
  gastrointestinal, and hypomagnesemia, 149
  intestinal, and hypokalemia, 133, 134, 139
  pancreatic, and hyponatremia, 122
Flaccid paralysis, 135
  and hyperkalemia, 141
Flaccidity and magnesium infusion, 155, 156
Fluid(s); see also Body fluid(s); Water
  extracellular; see Extracellular body fluid
  infusion of, 94–104; see also Intravenous fluids
    dangers with, 95
  intake of, 91, 93
  intake-output record of, 108, 109, 126
    in acid-base imbalance, 75

Fluids—cont'd
  intravenous, rate of administration of, 96
  maintenance, in children, calculation of,
    29
  oral, for hyponatremia, 122
  output of, per day, 91–92
  rate of flow of
    adjusting, 101–103
    calculation of, 98–99
    mechanical factors affecting, 100
  requirements for, 91–94
    for adults, 91–92
    for children, 92–94
    in elderly, 94
    for infants, 93
  restrictions on, 108
Fluid compartments
  interstitial, 3
  intracellular, 3
  intravascular, 3
Fluid and electrolyte balance, 1–42
Fluid and electrolyte imbalance, 39–42
Fluid compartments, 2–4
  electrolyte composition of, 12–14
Fluid volume; see Body fluid(s), volume of
Flushing
  from hypermagnesemia, 159
  during magnesium infusion, 155, 156
Fontanel
  anterior, palpating, 89
  and dehydration, 88
Foods
  rich in potassium, 136–137
  water from, 28
Force, filtration, 24
  net, 24
Foreign objects in airway causing respira-
    tory acidosis, 68
Fracture, pathological
  and osteoporosis, 169
  protection from, 177
Furosemide
  for hypercalcemia, 177
  and hypokalemia, 134

G

Gastric suction
  and chloride loss, 62
  and hypokalemia, 133, 134, 139

Gastrointestinal drainage
  and body fluid loss, 92
  and hyponatremia, 118
Gastrointestinal excretion of calcium, 164
Gastrointestinal fistula and hypomagnese-
    mia, 149
Gastrointestinal tract
  body fluid and, 5, 30, 82
  and potassium loss, 133
  and sodium balance, 116
Glucose
  5%, 18
  hypertonic, for hyperkalemia, 142–143
  intravenous administration of, 102
  metabolism of, 102–103
  in solution, 6
Glycosuria, 102
Gradient, pressure, 23
  hydrostatic, 24
  oncotic, 24
  osmotic, 28
Gravity, specific; see Specific gravity

H

Hallucinations
  in hypocalcemia, 168
  and hypomagnesemia, 152, 156
HCO_3^-, 66
Headache
  from metabolic acidosis, 71
  and sodium deficit, 119
Heart
  arrhythmia of, in respiratory alkalosis, 70
  effects of hypercalcemia on, 175
  hyperkalemia and, 141
  irregular rhythm of, and hypokalemia,
    135–136
Heart block
  from hyperkalemia, 141
  and hypokalemia, 135–136
Heart failure
  congestive, 25
    and hypernatremia, 124
    from infusion of fluid, 95–96
    symptoms of, 96, 107
  and edema of abdominal cavity, 125
  and excess body fluids, 105
  and hypernatremia, 124
  and pulmonary edema, 25–26, 125

Heart failure—cont'd
  severe, and fluid volume excess, 105
Heart rate in hypovolemia, 111–112
Hematocrit
  body fluid volume relationship to, 83
  in children, 84
  elevated, 83
  and fluid volume excess, 107
  hyponatremia and, 121
  normal, 83
Hemiplegia and fluid volume excess, 107–
    108
Hemodialysis
  for hyperkalemia, 143
  and hypocalcemia, 170
Hemoglobin buffer system, 51
Hemoglobin level, fluid volume excess and,
    107
Homeostasis, 35–36
  of hydrogen ion concentration, 43
  maintenance of, 35
  of water volume in body, 36
Hormone(s)
  adrenal cortical steroid, and potassium
    excretion, 134
  antidiuretic, and fluid volume regulation,
    36, 37, 38–39
  parathyroid
    magnesium and, 146–147
    and serum calcium, 164, 165
  parathyroid-like, and hypercalcemia, 173
  secretion of, calcium and, 163
Hydration for hypercalcemia, 176
Hydrochloric acid, 44, 50
  as buffer, 50
  loss of, causing metabolic alkalosis, 73
Hydrogen ions, 44, 45
  acceptor of, 44
  and bicarbonate ions, balance of, 53
  concentration of, 43–48; see also pH
    and potassium, 130
    and potassium control, 130
    and respiratory system, 52
  donor of, 44
  excretion of, by renal system, 52–53
Hydrostatic pressure, 22–23, 27, 34
  at arterial end of capillary, 24
  and oncotic pressure, 24
  at venous end of capillary, 24

Hydrostatic pressure gradient, 24
Hydroxyl ions, 45
Hyperactive breathing, 61, 62
Hyperactive reflexes and hypocalcemia,
    167–168
Hyperalimentation
  and hypocalcemia, 170
  and hypomagnesemia, 148–149
Hypercalcemia, 172–179
  causes of, 172–175
  and hypernatremia, 176
  and hyperparathyroidism, 173
  and hypokalemia, 176
  and hypomagnesemia, 150, 176
  signs and symptoms of, 174–176
  treatment of, 176–178
Hypercalcemic crisis, 176
Hyperkalemia, 139–144
  causes of, 139–141, 144
  changes in electrocardiograph from, 141–
    142
  and hypokalemia, 141
  intravenous administration of potassium-
    containing solutions causing, 140
  laboratory findings in, 142
  neuromuscular symptoms of, 141
  treatment of, 142–143
Hypermagnesemia, 158–161
  nursing considerations in, 160
  signs and symptoms of, 159–160
  treatment of, 144
Hypernatremia, 124–128
  causes of, 124
  and hypercalcemia, 176
  symptoms of, 125
  treatment of, 125–127
  and water retention, 125–126
Hyperparathyroidism, 153
  and hypercalcemia, 173
  primary, and hypomagnesemia, 150
Hyperphosphatemia and hypocalcemia, 167
Hyperpotassemia; see Hyperkalemia
Hypertonic dehydration, 87
  physical signs of, 88
Hypertonic glucose for hyperkalemia, 142–
    143
Hypertonic solution, 19
  for fluid volume excess, 108
  intravenous administration of, 102

Hypertrophic pyloric stenosis, 77–78
Hyperventilation causing respiratory alka-
    losis, 70
Hypocalcemia, 166–172
  causes of, 166–167
  and hyperphosphatemia, 167
  and hypomagnesemia, 152, 167
  mental changes in, 168
  nursing action in, 171, 172
  signs and symptoms of, 167–169
  treatment of, 170–171
Hypokalemia, 132–139
  and alkalosis, 132
  and hypercalcemia, 176
  and hyperkalemia, 141
  and serum potassium level, 136
  signs and symptoms of, 134–136, 139
    cardiac, 135–136
    gastrointestinal, 135
    neuromuscular, 134–135
  treatment of, 136–138
Hypomagnesemia, 148–158
  cardiovascular signs of, 152
  causes of, 148–149
  and hypercalcemia, 176
  and hypocalcemia, 152, 167
  neuromuscular signs of, 151–152
  nursing considerations in, 155–156
  signs and symptoms of, 151–153
  treatment of, 153–156
Hyponatremia, 118–122
  causes of, 118
  hematocrit level in, 121
  intravenous treatment of, 121–122
  laboratory findings in, 121
  serum levels in, 121
  signs and symptoms of, 119–121
  treatment of, 121–122
  urinary volume in, 121
Hypoparathyroidism and hypocalcemia, 166,
    167
Hypopotassemia; see Hypokalemia
Hypotension
  from hypermagnesemia, 144, 159
  and hypokalemia, 135–136
  and hypomagnesemia, 152
  during magnesium infusion, 155, 156
  orthostatic, and hyponatremia, 120
  from sodium deficit, 119

Hypothalamus and thirst stimulation, 35, 85
Hypotonic dehydration, 87
  physical signs of, 88
Hypotonic solution, 18–19, 26–27
  intravenous administration of, 102
  and swelling of cells, 19
Hypovolemia, 111–112
  clinical signs of, 111

I

Ileus, paralytic, and hypokalemia, 135
Immobilization, prolonged, and hypercal-
    cemia, 174
Infant
  dehydration in, 87–89
  fluid balance in, 1
  fluid requirements for, 93
  and fluid volume deficit, 84
  and fluid volume imbalance, 81–82
  infusion rates for, 97
  Signs of fluid deficit in, 91
Infection(s)
  and antidiuretic hormone secretion, 104
  urinary tract, and hypercalcemia, 178
Inflammation and fluid volume shift, 111,
    112
Infusion
  dangers of, 95
  fluids by, 94–104; see also Intravenous
    fluids
  of magnesium sulfate, 153–156
Inherited intestinal defects in magnesium
    absorption, 149
Injections, intramuscular, of magnesium
    sulfate, 153
Injury
  crush, and hyperkalemia, 140
  protecting patient from, 74–75
Insensible perspiration, 29
Insensible water loss, 30
Insulin
  and diabetic acidosis, 61
  as example of active transport, 21
  for hyperkalemia, 142–143
Intake and output recording, 108, 109
  in acid-base imbalance, 75
  in treatment of hypernatremia, 126
Interstitial body fluid, 3, 14
  electrolyte composition of, 13

Interstitial space, shift of fluids to, 110–112
Intestinal absorption, impaired, of magnesium, 149
Intestinal defects, inherited, in magnesium absorption, 149
Intestinal fistulas and hypokalemia, 133, 134, 139
Intestine, small, disease of, and hypocalcemia, 166, 167
Intracellular body fluid, 2–4, 14
    electrolyte composition of, 13
    osmotic balance of, with extracellular fluid, 84–85
    pH of, 47
    potassium as cation in, 129
    volume of, potassium in control of, 129–130
Intracellular compartment, 2, 3, 4
Intracranial lesions causing respiratory alkalosis, 70
Intramuscular injections of magnesium sulfate, 153
Intravascular body fluid, 2–3, 14
    electrolyte composition of, 13
    potassium in, 129–130
    shift of, into interstitial space, 110–112
Intravenous administration of normal saline for hypercalcemia, 176–177
Intravenous fluids; see also Fluid(s), infusion of
    administration sets for, 98
    drop size of, 98–99
    for hyponatremia, 121–122
    rate of administration of, 96
        adjusting, 101–103
        calculating, 98–99
        mechanical factors affecting, 100
    urinary output and, 102–103
Intravenous infusion
    of magnesium sulfate, 153–156
    of potassium, 137
    supervision of, 101
Intravenous solution, calcium in, 167
Ion(s), 7–8
    availability of, 10–11
    bicarbonate, and hydrogen ion balance, 53
    charge of, 7
    determining availability of, 10
    dissociation of electrolytes into, 8

Ion(s)—cont'd
    hydrogen; see Hydrogen ions
    hydroxyl, 45
    negatively charged, 7–8
    positively charged, 7
Ionized calcium, 161–162
Irritability, neuromuscular, and hypomagnesemia, 151–152
Iso-, 17
Isotonic dehydration, 87, 88
    physical signs of, 88
Isotonic saline solution, 18
    for hyponatremia, 121–122
Isotonic solutions, 17–18, 26, 27
    intravenous administration of, 102
    parenteral administration of, 94–95

K

Kaon; see potassium gluconate
Ketoacidosis, diabetic
    and hypermagnesemia, 159
    and hypomagnesemia, 150
Kidney
    and antidiuretic hormone, 83
    decreased blood flow through, and fluid volume excess, 104
    disease of
        and fluid volume excess, 104
        and hypercalcemia, 174
        and hypokalemia, 133–134
        and hypomagnesemia, 150
        and water deficit, 85
    excretion of body fluid by, 5, 82
    excretion of calcium by, 164
    excretion of hydrogen ions by, 54–55
    and extracellular fluid volume, 36
    and fluid and electrolyte balance, 30–31
    and fluid regulation, 42
    and hypokalemia, 135
    and magnesium, 146
    and magnesium conservation, 148
    pH balance and, 48, 52–55
    reaction of, to pH changes, 55
    respiratory acidosis compensation by, 57
    in respiratory alkalosis, 59
    and sodium balance, 116
    and sodium resorption, 124
Kidney stones from hypercalcemia, 175–176
Kussmaul breathing, 61, 62

L

Lactate-containing solutions
  for metabolic acidosis, 72
  for metabolic alkalosis, 73
  for respiratory acidosis, 70
Lasix; *see* Furosemide
Lassitude and sodium loss, 119
Law of osmosis, 82
Lesions
  cerebral, and antidiuretic hormone secretion, 105
  intracranial, causing respiratory alkalosis, 70
Lethargy and hypercalcemia, 174–175
Levophed; *see* Norepinephrine
Liquids, oral, water from, 5, 28
Liter, 9
Liver capillaries, 25
Liver cirrhosis
  and edema of abdominal cavity, 125
  and fluid volume excess, 105
  and hypernatremia, 124, 125
Lungs
  body fluid loss through, 5, 82
  cancer of, and antidiuretic hormone secretion, 105
  disease of, chronic obstructive, 79; *see also* Emphysema
  water loss through, 30, 85
Lymphatic blockage and fluid volume shift, 111
Lymphatics carrying protein, 25

M

Magnesium
  absorption of, 147
  and calcium, 146
  conservation of, 148
  deficit of, 148–158; *see also* Hypomagnesemia
  excess of, 158–161; *see also* Hypermagnesemia
  excessive loss of, 149–150
  functions of, 146
  imbalance of, 145–161
  ingestion of, amount of, 147
  normal levels of, 145
  sources of, 147
Magnesium bicarbonate, 49

Magnesium salts for hypomagnesemia, 153–156
Magnesium sulfate for hypomagnesemia, 153–156
Magnesium-containing medications causing hypermagnesemia, 158–159
Maintenance fluids in children, calculation of, 29
Malabsorption syndrome and hypomagnesemia, 149
Malaise from metabolic acidoisis, 71
Malignant tumors and hypercalcemia, 163
Malnutrition and hypomagnesemia, 148
Mask inhalation of carbon dioxide for respiratory alkalosis, 59, 60
Mean corpuscular volume and fluid volume excess, 107
Measurement of electrolytes, 9–11
Mechanical ventilation, 58
  for respiratory acidosis, 69
Medications, magnesium-containing, and hypermagnesemia, 158–159
Membrane; *see* Cell membranes; Mucous membranes
Memory, impairment of
  and hypercalcemia, 175
  in hypocalcemia, 168
Mental confusion and hypokalemia, 135; *see also* Confusion
Meperidine hydrochloride and antidiuretic hormone secretion, 105
Metabolic acidosis, 60–62, 77
  carbon dioxide content in, 67
  case study of, 78
  compensated, 72
  and hyperkalemia, 140, 142
  nursing care in, 71–73
  signs and symptoms of, 71
  summary of, 77
  treatment of, 61
  uncompensated, 72
Metabolic alkalosis, 62–63, 65
  case study of, 77–78
  and hypokalemia, 132–133, 136
  nursing care for, 73
  summary of, 63, 76
Metabolism as source of water, 5
Metaraminol for hyponatremia, 121
Metastasis, osteolytic, neoplastic disease with, 153

Milliequivalent, 10–11, 34
Milliliter, 9
Milliosmole, 20
Mithracin; *see* Mithramycin
Mithramycin for hypercalcemia, 177
Molecule, 6
Mood changes in hypocalcemia, 168
Morphine and antidiuretic hormone secretion, 105
Mucous membranes
  and fluid volume deficit, 85–86
  and hypernatremia, 125
Muscle(s), transmission of impulses in
  potassium and, 129–130
  sodium and, 115, 116
Muscle cramps
  and hypocalcemia, 167
  and hypokalemia, 135
  and sodium deficit, 119
Muscle paralysis and hyperkalemia, 141
Muscle tone, loss of, and hypercalcemia,
    174
Muscle weakness
  and hypercalcemia, 174
  and hypokalemia, 135, 139
  and sodium, 116
  and sodium deficit, 119
Myocardium and hyperkalemia, 140–141

N

Na; *see* Sodium
Nasogastric suction tube, 40
Nausea
  and hypercalcemia, 175
  in hypercalcemic crisis, 176
  from metabolic acidosis, 71
  and sodium deficit, 119
Neck veins, collapsed, in hyponatremia, 120
Needle, position of, and flow rate, 100
Neoplastic diseases
  and hypocalcemia, 167
  with metastasis to bone, 153
Nephritis
  potassium-losing, and hypokalemia, 133–
    134
  salt-losing, and hyponatremia, 118
Nerve cell membranes, excitability of, and
    calcium, 163

Nerve tissue, excitability of, and calcium,
    163
Nerves, transmission of impulses in
  calcium and, 163
  potassium and, 129–130
  sodium and, 115, 116
Net, 18
Net filtration force, 24
Net fluid shift, 18
Neural excitability and hypocalcemia, 167
Neuromuscular excitability, calcium and,
    163
Neuromuscular functions and magnesium,
    146, 147
Neuromuscular irritability
  and electrolytes, 115
  and hypomagnesemia, 151–152
  and potassium, 129–130
Neutral solution, 45
Neutron, 6
  charge of, 6
  position of, in atom, 6
Nontropical sprue and hypomagnesemia,
    149
Norepinephrine for hyponatremia, 121
Normal saline solution, 18
  for hypercalcemia, 176–177
"Nothing by mouth," 39–40
Nucleic acids, synthesis of, and magnesium, 146, 147
Nucleus of atom, 6
Numbness
  and hyperkalemia, 141
  and hypocalcemia, 167
Nurse, responsibility of, in administration of
    fluids, 95-97
Nursing care in acid-base imbalance, 66–
    77
Nutrients, body fluid transportation of, 2
Nutrition, total parenteral
  and hypocalcemia, 170
  and hypomagnesemia, 148–159

O

Obstructive lung disease, chronic, 79
Oliguria from potassium supplementation,
    137
Oncotic pressure, 23
  and hydrostatic pressure, 24

Oncotic pressure gradient, 24
Oral fluids for hyponatremia, 122
Orthostatic hypotension and hyponatremia, 120
Osmolality, 20–21, 27
   of plasma, normal, 21
Osmolarity, 20
   of body fluid and electrolytes, 15
Osmole, 20
Osmoreceptors, response of, to excess fluid, 104
Osmosis, 16–17, 26, 34
   law of, 82
   and movement of fluids, 129
Osmotic balance of extracellular and intra-
      cellular body fluids, 84–85
Osmotic equilibrium, 18
Osmotic force, 25
Osmotic pressure, 17, 26–27
   and ADH production, 39
   at arterial end of capillary, 24
   colloid, 23
      and hydrostatic pressure, 24
   and thirst initiation, 83
   at venous end of capillary, 24–25
Osmotic pressure gradient, 28
Osmotic pull; see Osmolarity
Osteolytic metastases, neoplastic disease
      with, 153
Osteoporosis, 169
Output and intake recording, 108, 109
   in acid-base imbalance, 75
   in treatment of hypernatremia, 126
Overhydration, 90
Oxidation
   of foods, water from, 28
   water of, 5
Oxygen tension, arterial, 66
Oxygen therapy for respiratory acidosis, 70
Oxytocin and fluid volume excess, 105

P

P wave and hyperkalemia, 141, 142
Pain
   abdominal, from metabolic acidosis, 71
   and antidiuretic hormone secretion, 104
   bone, deep, and hypercalcemia, 175
Palpitations in respiratory alkalosis, 70

Pancreatic disease and hypocalcemia, 166, 167
Pancreatic drainage and sodium loss, 128
Pancreatic fistula, sodium loss due to, 122
Paralysis
   flaccid
      and hyperkalemia, 141
      and hypokalemia, 135
      and hypokalemia, 139
   respiratory
      and hyperkalemia, 141
      during magnesium infusion, 155
Paralytic ileus and hypokalemia, 135
Parathyroid glands
   adenoma of, and hypercalcemia, 173
   surgery involving, hypocalcemia and, 170
Parathyroid hormone
   deficiency of, and hypocalcemia, 166, 167
   functions of, 165
   magnesium and, 146–147
   and serum calcium, 164, 165
Parathyroid-like hormone and hypercal-
      cemia, 173
Parenteral hyperalimentation and hypo-
      magnesemia, 148–149
Parenteral replacement for hyponatremia, 121–122
Paresthesias
   and hyperkalemia,141
   and hypocalcemia, 167
   and hypomagnesemia, 151
   and metabolic alkalosis, 73
Patellar reflex, loss of, and magnesium in-
      fusion, 155, 156
Pathological fracture
   and osteoporosis, 169
   protection from, 177
PCO_2
   changes in, 66, 67
   level of
      in metabolic acidosis, 72
      in respiratory acidosis, 69
      in respiratory alkalosis, 71
   range of, 66
Peptic ulcer disease and hypercalcemia, 172
Peripheral nervous system, excitation of, in
      alkalosis, 64
Peripheral pulse rate in hyponatremia, 120
Peristalsis, absent, and hypokalemia, 135

Peritoneal dialysis for hyperkalemia, 143
Peritonitis
    and hyponatremia, 118
    and sodium deficit, 123
Permeability
    of capillary walls, 25
    of cell membranes, 14
        and calcium, 163
    selective, 14, 15
Permeable cell membrane, 15, 16
Personality changes
    from hypercalcemia, 175
    with hypomagnesemia, 152
Perspiration, 30
    and fluid requirements, 92
    and hyponatremia, 118
    insensible, 29
    and respiratory alkalosis, 70
pH, 43, 47
    arterial, range of, 66
    as indicator of acidosis or alkalosis, 67
    limits of, in body fluid, 45
    measurement of, 66
    in metabolic acidosis, 72
    in metabolic alkalosis, 73
    normal range for, 45
    regulation of
        by buffer system, 50–51
        by renal system, 52–55
        by respiratory system, 52
    in respiratory acidosis, 69
    in respiratory alkalosis, 71
    use of symbol, 43
Phonation, muscles of, and hyperkalemia,
        141
Phosphate
    calcium and, 164, 165
    for hypercalcemia, 177
Phosphate buffer system, 51
Pituitary gland
    posterior
        and antidiuretic hormone secretion, 83
        and fluid volume excess, 104
        and sodium balance, 116
        and urine volume regulation, 83
Plasma
    normal osmolality of, 21
    rapid dilution of, and hypocalcemia, 167
Pneumonia causing respiratory acidosis , 68

PO_2, 66
    range of, 66
Poisoning, salicylate, respiratory alkalosis
        from, 58–59
Polarization and hyperkalemia, 141
Polyuria from hypercalcemia, 175
Posterior pituitary gland
    and antidiuretic hormone secretion, 83
    and fluid volume excess, 104
Potassium
    as cation of intracellular fluid, 33
    deficit of, 132–139; see also Hypokalemia
        causes of, 133
        oral replacement of, 136–137
        range of, 137
    electrical charge of, 130
    excess of, 139–144; see also Hyperkalemia
    excretion of, 131
        and magnesium, 146
        regulation of, 131–132
    filtered, 131
    foods rich in, 136–137
    function of, in body, 129
    imbalance in, 128–145
        signs and symptoms of, 130
    intake of, 133
    and intracellular fluid volume, 129–130
    intravenous administration of, 137–138
        causing hyperkalemia, 140
    level of
        alkalosis and, 132
        serum
            low; see Hypokalemia
            normal, 129
    loss of, 11
    and neuromuscular irritability, 129–130
    and osmosis, 129
    replacement of, 41–42, 136–137
    resorption of, 131
    serum level of
        in hyponatremia, 121
        normal, 136
    sources of, 136–137
    supplementation of, 133
    and transmission of electrochemical im-
        pulses, 129–130
Potassium bicarbonate, 49
Potassium chloride
    as hypokalemia treatment, 137

Sodium—cont'd
  serum, and hyponatremia, 121
  and transmission of impulses, 115–116, 129
  in urine, 116
Sodium bicarbonate, 49
  for diabetic acidosis, 61
  formation of, 50
  for hyperkalemia, 142–143
  for metabolic acidosis, 72
Sodium chloride
  dissociation of, 6, 8, 9
  intravenous administration of, 122
  resorbed sodium in, 116
  and sodium deficit, 119
  0.85% solution, 18
  10% solution, 19
Sodium hydroxide as buffer, 50
Sodium lactate for diabetic acidosis, 61
Sodium-potassium ratio, 130
Solute, 14, 15
Solution
  acidic, 44, 45
  alkaline, 44, 45
  chloride-containing, for metabolic alkalosis, 63, 73
  hypertonic; see Hypertonic solution
  hypotonic; see Hypotonic solution
  intravenous, calcium in, 167
  isotonic; see Isotonic solutions
  lactate-containing, for metabolic acidosis, 72
  neutral, 45
  osmolality of, 21
  pH of, 44
  saline; see Saline solution
Solvent, 15
Spasm
  carpal, and hypocalcemia, 168
  tonic, from alkalosis, 64
Specific gravity
  of body fluids, 20–21
  of urine
    and dehydration, 89
    normal, 84
Spironolactone for aldosterone overproduction, 127
Sprue, nontropical, and hypomagnesemia, 149

S-T segment and hypokalemia, 136
Standstill, ventricular, from hyperkalemia, 141
Starvation and hypomagnesemia, 148
Steatorrhea and hypomagnesemia, 149
Stenosis, pyloric, hypertrophic, 77–78
Steroid hormones, adrenal corticoid, and potassium excretion, 134
Stones, kidney, and hypercalcemia, 175–176
Stress, antidiuretic hormone secretion and, 105, 108
Strong acid, 44
Stupor
  and hypercalcemia, 175
  in hypercalcemic crisis, 176
Suction, gastric, and hypokalemia, 133, 134
Sulfuric acid, 44
Supplementation, potassium, 133
Surgery
  abdominal, and fluid volume shift, 110–111
  hypocalcemia after, 170
  hypomagnesemia after, 150
Swallowing, difficult, and water loss, 85
Sweating; see Perspiration
Swelling of cells, 19
Syndrome
  Cushing's, 38
  malabsorption, and hypomagnesemia, 149
  water-excess, 108

T
T wave
  in hypercalcemia, 175
  in hyperkalemia, 141, 142
  in hypokalemia, 136
  in hypomagnesemia, 152
Tachycardia
  and hypomagnesemia, 152
  and hyponatremia, 120
  ventricular, from calcium and digitalis, 170–171
Teeth, calcium in, 162–163
Temperature
  high; see Fever
  and water intake requirements, 92
Tension
  carbon dioxide, arterial, 66

Tension—cont'd
 oxygen, arterial, 66
Testosterone for hyperkalemia, 143
Tests indicating fluid volume deficit, 84
Tetany
 and alkalosis, 46, 64
 and hypocalcemia, 167, 172
 and hypomagnesemia, 151
 from metabolic alkalosis, 73
 in respiratory alkalosis, 70
Thiazides and hypokalemia, 134
Third spacing, 110–112, 113
Thirst, 83
 and fluid intake, 35–36
 impairment of sense of, 84–85
 as water deficit symptom, 84–85
Thyrocalcitonin and serum calcium, 164
Thyroid gland, surgery involving, hypocalcemia and, 170
Tingling sensations
 and hyperkalemia, 141
 and hypocalcemia, 167
 in respiratory alkalosis, 70
Tissue
 nerve, excitability of, and calcium, 163
 trauma to, and hyperkalemia, 140
Tongue
 changes in, in sodium deficit, 120
 and fluid volume deficit, 85–86
Tonic spasm from alkalosis, 64
Total parenteral nutrition
 and hypocalcemia, 170
 and hypomagnesemia, 148–149
Toxemia of pregnancy, magnesium and,
  146
Tracheostomy and water loss, 85
Trauma
 and fluid volume shift, 111
 to tissues and hyperkalemia, 140
Tremor and hypomagnesemia, 151
Triamterene, 134
Trousseau's sign and hypocalcemia, 168
Tube, nasogastric suction, 40
Tumors, malignant, and hypercalcemia, 163
Turgor, skin; see Skin turgor

U

U wave and hypokalemia, 136
Ulcer, peptic, 172

Uncompensated metabolic acidosis, 72
Unconsciousness
 from acid-base imbalance, 74
 from metabolic acidosis, 71
Units of measurement of body fluids, 9
Urea in solution, 6
Uremic acidosis causing metabolic acidosis,
  60
Ureteroenterostomy and hypokalemia, 133–
  134
Urinary output and fluid volume excess,
  104
Urinary tract
 infections of, and hypercalcemia, 178
 stones in, and hypercalcemia, 177–178
Urine
 acidic, 53
  to prevent stone formation, 178
 alkaline, 53, 59
 excretion of, antidiuretic hormone and,
  83
 glucose excreted in, 103
 loss of magnesium via, 148
 normal specific gravity of, 84
 output of, 31
  average values for, 92, 93
  and dehydration, 88–89
  and fluid intake, 91–92
  and hypercalcemia, 175
  and hyperkalemia, 140
  in hypernatremia, 125
  in hypokalemia, 133–134, 135
  in hyponatremia, 120
  in hypovolemia, 112
 potassium loss through, 133
 sodium in, 116
 volume of, regulation of, 36

V

Veins, neck, in hyponatremia, 120
Ventilation, mechanical, 58
 for respiratory acidosis, 69
Ventricular arrhythmias and hypercalcemia,
  175
Ventricular contraction, premature
 from calcium and digitalis, 170–171
 and hypomagnesemia, 152
Ventricular fibrillation from respiratory acidosis, 68

Ventricular standstill from hyperkalemia, 141
Ventricular tachycardia from calcium and digitalis, 170–171
Vertigo and sodium deficit, 119
Vital signs and acid-base imbalance, 74
Vitamin D
    actions of, 165
    and calcium, 164–165
    deficiency of, and hypocalcemia, 166, 167
    excessive, and hypercalcemia, 172, 173
    and serum calcium, 164
    sources of, 164
Vitamins, B, and magnesium, 146
Volume
    blood, and extracellular fluid volume, 36
    extracellular fluid, 36
    fluid; see Body fluid(s), volume of
Volume control device for intravenous infusion, 97, 98
Vomiting
    and body fluid loss, 1, 92
    and chloride loss, 62
    and hydrochloric acid loss, causing metabolic alkalosis, 73
    and hypercalcemia, 175
    and hypokalemia, 133, 134, 139
    and hyponatremia, 118, 119
    from metabolic acidosis, 71

W

Waste products, body fluid transportation of, 2
Water; see also Body fluid(s); Fluid(s)
    balance of, into and out of body, 31
    deficit of, 82
        severe, signs of, 86

Water—cont'd
    thirst as symptom of, 84–85
    distilled, 18–19
        oral intake of, 94
    drinking, 94
        to correct fluid volume deficit, 83
    and electrolytes entering and leaving body, normal mechanisms for, 28–32
    formation of, 45
        from buffer solution, 50
    intake of
        increasing, 94
        regulation of, 126
    loss of
        by diffusion through skin, 29, 30
        through expired air, 30
    of oxidation, 5
    retention of; see Edema
Water-excess syndrome, 108
Weak acid, 44
Weakness, muscle
    and hypercalcemia, 174
    and hyperkalemia, 126
    and hypokalemia, 139
    from metabolic acidosis, 71
    and respiratory acidosis, 68
    as sign of body water deficit, 86
    from sodium loss, 119
Weight
    changes in, as sign of dehydration, 88–89
    equivalent, 10
    fluid percentage of, 1, 4–5
    gain in, and fluid volume excess, 106
Weight record and hypernatremia treatment, 126
Wound exudate and fluid loss, 92